T0226417

Caring for the Geriatric Surgical Patient

Editor

FRED A. LUCHETTE

SURGICAL CLINICS
OF NORTH AMERICA

www.surgical.theclinics.com

Consulting Editor
RONALD F. MARTIN

February 2015 • Volume 95 • Number 1

ELSEVIER

1600 John F. Kennedy Boulevard • Suite 1800 • Philadelphia, Pennsylvania, 19103-2899

http://www.surgical.theclinics.com

SURGICAL CLINICS OF NORTH AMERICA Volume 95, Number 1
February 2015 ISSN 0039–6109, ISBN-13: 978-0-323-35451-6

Editor: John Vassallo, j.vassallo@elsevier.com
Developmental Editor: Colleen Viola

Surgical Clinics of North America (ISSN 0039–6109) is published bimonthly by Elsevier Inc., 360 Park Avenue South, New York, NY 10010-1710. Months of publication are February, April, June, August, October, and December. Business and Editorial Offices: 1600 John F. Kennedy Blvd., Suite 1800, Philadelphia, PA 19103-2899. Periodicals postage paid at New York, NY and additional mailing offices. Subscription prices are $370.00 per year for US individuals, $627.00 per year for US institutions, $180.00 per year for US students and residents, $455.00 per year for Canadian individuals, $793.00 per year for Canadian institutions, $510.00 for international individuals, $793.00 per year for international institutions and $250.00 per year for Canadian and foreign students/residents. To receive student/resident rate, orders must be accompanied by name of affiliated institution, date of term, and the *signature* of program/residency coordinator on institution letterhead. Orders will be billed at individual rate until proof of status is received. Foreign air speed delivery is included in all *Clinics* subscription prices. All prices are subject to change without notice. POSTMASTER: Send address changes to *Surgical Clinics*, Elsevier Health Sciences Division, Subscription Customer Service, 3251 Riverport Lane, Maryland Heights, MO 63043. **Customer Service (orders, claims, online, change of address): Telephone: 1-800-654-2452 (U.S. and Canada); 314-447-8871 (outside U.S. and Canada). Fax: 314-447-8029. E-mail: journalscustomerservice-usa@elsevier.com (for print support); journalsonline support-usa@elsevier.com (for online support).**

Reprints. For copies of 100 or more, of articles in this publication, please contact the Commercial Reprints Department, Elsevier Inc., 360 Park Avenue South, New York, New York 10010-1710. Tel. 212-633-3874, Fax: 212-633-3820, E-mail: reprints@elsevier.com.

The *Surgical Clinics of North America* is also published in Spanish by McGraw-Hill Interamericana Editores S.A., P.O. Box 5-237 06500 Mexico D.F. Mexico; and in Portuguese by Interlivros Edicoes Ltda., Rua Comandante Coelho 1085, CEP 21250, Rio de Janeiro, Brazil; and in Greek by Paschalidis Medical Publications, Athens Greece.

The *Surgical Clinics of North America* is covered in *MEDLINE/PubMed (Index Medicus)*, *EMBASE/Excerpta Medica*, *Current Contents/Clinical Medicine*, *Current Contents/Life Sciences*, *Science Citation Index*, and *ISI/BIOMED*.

Contributors

CONSULTING EDITOR

RONALD F. MARTIN, MD
Staff Surgeon, Department of Surgery, Marshfield Clinic, Marshfield, Wisconsin; Clinical Associate Professor, University of Wisconsin School of Medicine and Public Health, Madison, Wisconsin; Colonel, Medical Corps, United States Army Reserve

EDITOR

FRED A. LUCHETTE, MD, MSc, FACS, FCCM
Chief of Surgical Services, Edward J. Hines Jr. Veterans Medical Center, Vice-Chair, VA Affairs, Professor of Surgery, Department of Surgery, Stritch School of Medicine, Loyola University Chicago, Hines, Illinois

AUTHORS

SASHA D. ADAMS, MD, FACS
Assistant Professor of Surgery, Division of Acute Care Surgery, Department of Surgery, The University of North Carolina at Chapel Hill, Chapel Hill, North Carolina

HASAN B. ALAM, MD, FACS
Norman Thompson Professor of Surgery, Chief of General Surgery, Department of Surgery, University of Michigan Hospital, University of Michigan, Ann Arbor, Michigan

ANTHONY J. BALDEA, MD
Assistant Professor of Surgery, Division of Trauma, Critical Care and Burns, Loyola University Medical Center, Maywood, Illinois

SUSAN E. BIFFL, MD
Department of Orthopedic Surgery, Denver Health Medical Center; Assistant Professor of Physical Medicine and Rehabilitation, University of Colorado Denver School of Medicine, Denver, Colorado

WALTER L. BIFFL, MD
Associate Director of Surgery, Denver Health Medical Center; Professor of Surgery, University of Colorado Denver School of Medicine, Denver, Colorado

GRANT V. BOCHICCHIO, MD, MPH
Edison Professor of Surgery and Chief of Acute and Critical Care Surgery, Washington University in St. Louis School of Medicine, St. Louis, Missouri

KAREN J. BRASEL, MD, MPH
Department of Surgery, Oregon Health & Science University, Portland, Oregon

MICHAEL C. CHANG, MD
Professor of Surgery, Department of Surgery, Wake Forest School of Medicine, Winston-Salem, North Carolina

JAE S. CHO, MD, FACS
Chief, Vascular Surgery & Endovascular Therapy; Professor, Surgery and Cardiothoracic Surgery, Stritch School of Medicine, Loyola University Chicago, Maywood, Illinois

JASON P. FARRAH, MD
Assistant Professor of Surgery, Department of Surgery, University of South Florida College of Medicine, Tampa, Florida

DAVID G. GREENHALGH, MD, FACS
Professor and Chief of Burns, Department of Surgery, Shriners Hospitals for Children Northern California, University of California, Davis Medical Center, Sacramento, California

IHAB HALAWEISH, MD
Department of Surgery, University of Michigan, Ann Arbor, Michigan

HAYTHAM M.A. KAAFARANI, MD, MPH
Assistant Professor of Surgery, Division of Trauma, Emergency Surgery and Surgical Critical Care, Massachusetts General Hospital, Harvard Medical School, Boston, Massachusetts

R. SHAYN MARTIN, MD
Department of Surgery, Wake Forest School of Medicine, Winston-Salem, North Carolina

EDEN NOHRA, MD
Acute and Critical Care Surgery, Washington University in St. Louis School of Medicine, St. Louis, Missouri

ANDREW B. PEITZMAN, MD
Department of Surgery, University of Pittsburgh, Pittsburgh, Pennsylvania

JACOB PESCHMAN, MD
Department of Surgery, Medical College of Wisconsin, Milwaukee, Wisconsin

ELIE RAMLY, MD
Research Fellow, Division of Trauma, Emergency Surgery and Surgical Critical Care, Massachusetts General Hospital, Harvard Medical School, Boston, Massachusetts

PRESTON B. RICH, MD, MBA, FACS
Professor of Surgery and Chief, Division of Acute Care Surgery, Department of Surgery, The University of North Carolina at Chapel Hill, Chapel Hill, North Carolina

THOMAS M. SCALEA, MD, FACS, MCCM
Physician in Chief, R Adams Cowley Shock Trauma Center; System Chief for Critical Care Services, University of Maryland Medical System; Honorable Francis X Kelly Distinguished Professor in Trauma; Director, Program In Trauma, University of Maryland School of Medicine, Baltimore, Maryland

KAREN G. SCANDRETT, MD
Department of Geriatric Medicine, University of Pittsburgh, Pittsburgh, Pennsylvania

MARTIN A. SCHREIBER, MD, FACS
Professor of Surgery and Chief, Division of Trauma, Critical Care & Acute Care Surgery, Department of Surgery, Oregon Health & Science University, Portland, Oregon

JANINE THEN, PharmD
Adjunct Instructor, Department of Pharmacy and Therapeutics, University of Pittsburgh, Pittsburgh, Pennsylvania

JIDE TINUBU, MD
Assistant Professor, Department of Orthopedics, University of Maryland School of Medicine, Baltimore, Maryland

SAMUEL A. TISHERMAN, MD, FACS, FCCM
Professor, Department of Surgery, University of Maryland, Baltimore, Maryland

PHILBERT Y. VAN, MD
Assistant Professor of Surgery, Division of Trauma, Critical Care & Acute Care Surgery, Department of Surgery, Oregon Health & Science University, Portland, Oregon

GEORGE C. VELMAHOS, MD, PhD
Professor of Surgery; Chief, Division of Trauma, Emergency Surgery and Surgical Critical Care, Massachusetts General Hospital, Harvard Medical School, Boston, Massachusetts

ED VILLELLA, MD
Vascular Surgery Fellow, Loyola University Medical Center, Maywood, Illinois

BRIAN S. ZUCKERBRAUN, MD
VA Pittsburgh Healthcare System; Department of Surgery, University of Pittsburgh, Pittsburgh, Pennsylvania

Contents

continues to grow. Much is already known about the basic risk factors associated with vascular aging, but there is a new direction of investigation into the health and viability of the endothelium at a biochemical level. As we continue to shift much of our health care focus into prevention tactics and techniques, slowing or reversing the aging process of the vascular system could have a profound impact on our aging population.

such as malnutrition, diabetes mellitus, treatment of malignancies, and vascular disease, all impair tissue repair. The geriatric population is more prone to pressure ulcers, venous stasis ulcers, and other chronic wounds. This review discusses how changes in the elderly lead to impaired healing or chronic wounds. Prevention of these problems and their treatment are also discussed.

Trauma is an increasingly common problem in geriatric patients; fractures are frequent among the elderly. Life expectancy continues to rise. Advances in medical care allow people to live longer and better lives. Medications, surgical advances (treatment for coronary artery disease, coronary bypass grafting), and joint replacement surgery can be safely performed in elderly patients. Thus, geriatric patients are no longer confined to a life of inactivity. They are out of their homes and interacting in the community, exercising and leading active lives. Thus, they are more likely to become injured and present to trauma centers for care.

Geriatric patients are at higher risk for hemorrhagic complications after surgery and traumatic injuries. The geriatric population is more likely to take anticoagulant or antiplatelet medications. Chronic disease, autoimmune disease, and nutritional deficiencies can lead to coagulation factor and platelet disorders. One must be familiar with the current anticoagulant and antiplatelet medications, their mechanism of action, and reversal agents to properly care for this group of patients. The new oral anticoagulants do not have Food and Drug Administration (FDA) approved reversal agents, but known procoagulant agents with other FDA indications may be effective.

Alterations in pharmacokinetics and pharmacodynamics place geriatric patients at an increased risk of experiencing an adverse drug event. The incidence of medication-related adverse events can be decreased with careful selection of agents and appropriate dosage adjustments.

As the population ages, the health care system must to adapt to the needs of the older population. Hospitalization risks are particularly significant in the frail geriatric patients, with costly and morbid consequences. Appropriate preoperative assessment can identify sources of increased risk and enable the surgical team to manage this risk, through "prehabilitation," intraoperative modification, and postoperative care. Geriatric preoperative assessment expands usual risk stratification and careful medication

SURGICAL CLINICS
OF NORTH AMERICA

FORTHCOMING ISSUES

April 2015
Perioperative Management
Paul J. Schenarts, *Editor*

June 2015
Surgical Approaches to Esophageal Disease
Dmitry Oleynikov, *Editor*

August 2015
Simulation in Surgical Training and Practice
Kimberly M. Brown and John T. Paige,
Editors

RECENT ISSUES

December 2014
Surgical Infections
Robert G. Sawyer and Traci L. Hedrick,
Editors

October 2014
Melanoma
Kimberly M. Brown and Celia Chao,
Editors

August 2014
Management of Burns
Robert L. Sheridan, *Editor*

June 2014
Endocrine Surgery
Peter J. Mazzaglia, *Editor*

ISSUE OF RELATED INTEREST

Clinics in Geriatric Medicine
May 2014 (Vol. 30, Issue 2)
Fragility Fractures
Susan M. Friedman and Daniel Ari Mendelson, *Editors*

Foreword

Caring for Geriatric Surgical Patients

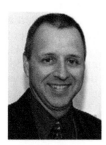

Ronald F. Martin, MD
Consulting Editor

It's tough to make predictions, especially about the future.
—*Lawrence Peter "Yogi" Berra*

From the time the Sumerian civilization began to form during the Uruk period, approximately four millennia BCE until fairly recently, the most medicine had to offer people to keep them alive and postpone death was not very much. Some people lived to become very old; some died very young, and most died earlier than they do in the present day. The probability curve for longevity of life was more centered.

Fast forward six thousand years, give or take, and we have developed an understanding of human anatomy, general anesthesia, the germ theory, antibiotics, organized medical training programs, cardiopulmonary bypass, the ability to ventilate and oxygenate via endotracheal means outside of an operating room, hemodialysis, solid organ transplantation, implantable hardware for repair of fractures and joint replacement, artificial heart valves, central venous access, total parenteral nutrition, new antibiotics to deal with organisms resistant to the old antibiotics, vasoactive agents, implantable cardioverter-defibrillators, and a whole host of other devices, drugs, procedures, and imaging devices. Yet, despite our profound advances in knowledge and technological sophistication, we did not necessarily develop the wisdom to know why we developed it or when not to use it.

Until the 1950s or 1960s, when someone told a doctor, "Do whatever you can, Doc," it was a pretty limited request, albeit not recognized as such. Today, the same request has very few limitations. There is certainly marked disparity between countries and cultures about how much health care is available, expected, or provided. There are clear differences in how people allocate and pay for health care. Nonetheless, one thing holds true across all types of health care systems: the better you get at dealing with problems that end life prematurely, the larger number of elderly people you get.

Surg Clin N Am 95 (2015) xiii–xv
http://dx.doi.org/10.1016/j.suc.2014.10.001
0039-6109/15/$ – see front matter © 2015 Published by Elsevier Inc.
surgical.theclinics.com

Of course, the ultrapurist can claim exception, such as China following its one-child policy. Then again, even China will catch up with the population distribution of the rest of the developed world. In the meantime, China will have a huge number of elderly people dependent on a relatively small number of young people. Still, since we are inherently mortal, the higher we push the average life expectancy, the closer we will get to people living as long as they can.

Although people live better and longer than they used to, there are still some inescapable consequences of aging. Dr Luchette and his colleagues have compiled a series of articles that outline these changes, system by system. Not only do all of our internal systems lose strength and reliability as we age, but we, as older people, are more likely to have one or more chronic diseases than younger people do. Although none of this may be surprising or appear other than just plain intuitive, we as a society, especially in the United States, still do not seem to grasp the implications of the tidal wave of challenges coming toward us.

All is not lost, though—quite the contrary. If we are to do well with this dilemma, there are some fundamental steps that must be taken. Primarily, we need to stop thinking about what we *can* do and focus on what we *should* do. More importantly, we need to know what our patients want us to do. Patients have different hopes, dreams, fears, and desires, and no matter how many guidelines or standards we establish, as doctors, hospitals, policy-makers, and regulators, we won't change those differences in desires—nor should we.

Second, we need to eliminate, or at least attenuate, the myopic obstacles to preventative care based on return on investment. If we have procedures or treatment practices that are expensive up-front, but cost effective in the long term (even though it may take a while to recover the initial investment), we should try our best to employ them. Conversely, if we are spending loads of money with no hope of recovery, then we need to reconsider that as well. At present, most patients do not spend their lifetime covered by one insurance plan (unless it is Medicare), and the turnover rate of carriers will inevitably lead to situations in which the cost of prevention will yield benefits that will be realized by another entity. This leads to suspension of services that may be valuable to the patient or even society—just not to the insurance carrier of the moment. Any number of schemes could be created to offset these displaced risks, but we haven't done that yet.

Third, we need to remove, or at least substantially degrade, the conflict of interest generated by pay for utilization and consumption. Although no rational person wants to reward people for "doing nothing," we must be able to not penalize people for doing the right thing when doing less or nothing is in the patient's best interest. If we incent utilization, we increase utilization. Virtually all schemes for which we have tried to "voluntarily" destroy demand have failed miserably over the past 30 years or so. The last few years, however, have seen demand destruction on an unprecedented scale. However, I fear that may not be entirely good news. High-deductible insurance plans have caused patients to seek and utilize health care more as if they are uninsured than as if they are in a "free-market" economy. Although the temporary decrease in demand has been enough to bend the projected cost curve downward, we are probably not at a position in which we can intelligently say whether there will be a more expensive deflection later due to inappropriately deferred care.

One article in this volume to which I specifically refer the reader is by Drs Rich and Adams on the economics of health care for the elderly. It is an excellent summary of the broad concepts that we, as surgeons, must understand to function not only within the health system but also within our communities. Respectfully, some of the predictions that they report appear dubious to me (not because of the authors, but because of the sources), but even if those predictions are completely wrong, their analysis of the system is still fundamental. And, in fairness, a financial prediction modeled out to the year 2080 has a very slim chance of holding up.

Every economic model of medicine shows improved performance if one can do things better, faster, and cheaper, with fewer complications. But money isn't everything. We must also ensure that we are, to the best of our ability, actually helping our patients live the lives they wish to lead. We need to do better what many of us now do quite poorly—ask patients what sort of limits they want to put on us and what goals they really have. We need to truly educate our patients about what their problems and their options are. We need to do this in such a way that we do not put our interests and priorities ahead of their interests and priorities. In short, we need to give them the tools to help assure their best possible futures. And, as Mr Berra tells us, when it comes to making predictions, predictions about the future are tough.

Last, even if you are not inclined to think this collection of articles is useful in your practice at present, with luck it may be information you need for yourself one day as a patient—if you live long enough. Enjoy.

Ronald F. Martin, MD
Department of Surgery
Marshfield Clinic
1000 North Oak Avenue
Marshfield, WI 54449, USA

E-mail address:
Martin.ronald@marshfieldclinics.org

Preface

Caring for the Geriatric Surgical Patient

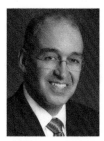

Fred A. Luchette, MD, MSc, FACS, FCCM
Editor

Since 1950, the United States has been in the midst of a profound demographic change: rapid aging of the population. This is in large part due to the advances in medical research that have resulted in new therapies for diseases, allowing humans to enjoy living longer than in the history of mankind. Life expectancy in the United States has improved dramatically over the past century—from 47.3 years in 1900 to 78.1 years in 2008. Finally, the number of persons aged 65 and older was 35.1 million in 2000, which was 12.4% of the population. By 2050, this group will reach 20.2% or 85.5 million.

The medical community is now just beginning to unravel and understand the effect of aging on organ function and the cumulative effect on the patient. Considering increased comorbidities and distinctly different physiologic responses/reserves, the geriatric patient will continue to present an array of challenges for all aspects of health care management. With surgeons being asked to care for these elderly patients, it is apparent that they are versed with the unique physiologic nuances that accompany the primary diagnosis.

In this issue of *Surgical Clinics of North America*, many established, highly accomplished luminaries in Acute Care Surgery have contributed their knowledge and expertise. We begin with the changing demographics of America, review the effect of aging on each organ system, and conclude with difficult end-of-life decisions that are relevant when caring for the elderly.

I applaud the editors for recognizing the importance of the elderly surgical patients that are presenting for surgical care. This is the first issue published on this topic in *Surgical Clinics of North America*. It has been a special honor for me to put this issue together. I want to specifically thank the editors for the confidence in me, the editorial

Surg Clin N Am 95 (2015) xvii–xviii
http://dx.doi.org/10.1016/j.suc.2014.09.018
0039-6109/15/$ – see front matter Published by Elsevier Inc.

surgical.theclinics.com

staff for their assistance, and the authors for giving of their time and expertise. I am confident that surgeons will find this issue informative and relevant to their practice.

Fred A. Luchette, MD, MSc, FACS, FCCM
Edward J. Hines Jr Veterans Medical Center
Department of Surgery
Stritch School of Medicine
Loyola University of Chicago
5000 South 5th Avenue
Hines, IL 60141, USA

E-mail addresses:
Frederick.luchette@va.gov, fluchet@lumc.edu

Changing Demographics of the American Population

Ihab Halaweish, MD, Hasan B. Alam, MD*

KEYWORDS

- Geriatric • Demographics • United States

KEY POINTS

- Currently in the United States, 1 in 9 Americans is aged 65 years or older; by 2050, this will increase to 1 in 5 Americans.
- The distribution of men and women who are older than 85 years—the oldest-old—will increase substantially by 2050.
- The prevalence and severity of comorbidity—the co-occurrence of multiple chronic conditions—will also increase.
- Life expectancy at 65 years of age has increased more in the past 30 years than in the entire 200-year period from 1750 to 1950; today, a person aged 65 years can expect to live another 15 years.
- Mortality from cardiac disease and stroke has decreased during the past 2 decades, whereas deaths from diabetes-related complications and Alzheimer disease are increasing.
- The aging of the population will have wide-ranging implications for the health care system.

INTRODUCTION

As noted by the Population Reference Bureau, "The U.S. is getting bigger, older, and more diverse." Since 1950, the United States has been in the midst of a profound demographic change: the rapid aging of the population. The baby boom generation began turning 65 in 2011 and is now driving growth at the older ages of the population.[1] This report highlights geriatric demographic changes and illustrates how these and future trends will have wide-ranging implications for the US health care system.

DEMOGRAPHIC TRENDS
Baby Boom Generation

In the post–World War II era, Americans started families at younger ages and in greater percentages than during the Great Depression. Between 1946 and 1964, this resulted

Department of Surgery, University of Michigan Hospital, University of Michigan, 2920 Taubman Center/5331, 1500 East Medical Center Drive, Ann Arbor, MI 48109-5331, USA
* Corresponding author.
E-mail address: alamh@med.umich.edu

Surg Clin N Am 95 (2015) 1–10
http://dx.doi.org/10.1016/j.suc.2014.09.002
0039-6109/15/$ – see front matter © 2015 Elsevier Inc. All rights reserved.
surgical.theclinics.com

in a surge in births and increased family sizes.[2] In 2000, the US population was typical of one experiencing slow growth. The population has been aging as life expectancy has increased markedly.[2] The number of persons aged 65 years and older reached 35.1 million in 2000, representing 12.4% of the US population, an increase from 8.1% in 1950. By 2050, the older population will reach 20.2%, around 88.5 million. In other words, 1 in 5 persons in 2050 will be aged 65 years or older.

Fig. 1 illustrates the importance of the baby boom generation in shaping the overall population demographics. In 2010, the baby boom generation was 46 to 64 years old. The 2010 population pyramid for the age groups near 20 years is a result of children born to baby boomers. All of the baby boomers will have moved into the ranks of the older population by 2030, resulting in a shift in the age structure, from 13% of the population aged 65 years and older in 2010 to 19% in 2030. Even after the youngest of the baby boom population have passed away, aging will continue to be one of the most important defining characteristics of the US population, reflecting continuing low fertility and improving survival in the United States.[1]

Age Composition

Half of women and almost three-fifths of men in the United States aged 65 years and older are in the 65- to 74-year age group, and one-third of both men and women are aged 75 to 84 years, whereas only one-tenth of men and one-sixth of women are aged 85 years or older. Between 2009 and 2030, this age distribution of the older population will remain mostly unchanged; however, by 2050 significant changes are expected: the distribution of men and women who are aged 85 years and older—the oldest-old—will increase substantially, whereas the shares of both men and women in the youngest age group will decline. Almost one-quarter of all women and one-fifth of all men aged 65 years and older will be in the oldest-old group. Given that the oldest-old have the highest rates of disability and institutionalization, this demographic shift will place significant strains on the state and federal budgets.[3]

Gender Changes

In the future, women will continue to constitute most of the older population, because women live longer than men in the United States; however, the difference between male and female life expectancy at birth has been decreasing. In 1979, this difference peaked at 7.8 years and decreased to 5.0 years in 2008. As people age, this gap shrinks, with men having a life expectancy of 17.0 years at age 65 years, whereas women's life expectancy at age 65 years is 19.7 years—a gap of less than 3 years. This gap decreases to only 1 year by age of 85.[3]

Ethnic Changes

In addition to disparities between men and women regarding aging, disparities exist between blacks and whites. White men in the United States on average have a life expectancy of 29 years and white women of 33 years at age 50 years.[4] Older black men and women, however, may not expect to live as long at the age of 50, with life expectancies of 25 and 30 years, respectively. Since the 1970s, the black/white gap in male life expectancy at age 50 years has remained longer than it was since 1930, but signs indicate that this gap is starting to narrow again.[5] The current racial gap in life expectancy at older ages for men may largely be attributed to trends in heart disease among men in the 60 years and older age group. From the 1970s through the 1990s, blacks experienced a slower decline in mortality from heart disease than whites. Recent evidence from analysis of the black/white life expectancy gap suggests a decline in

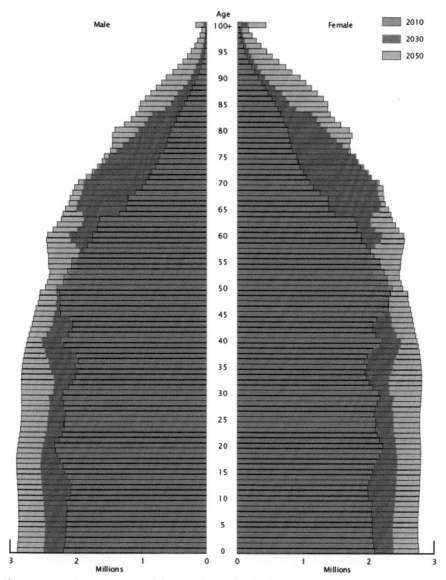

Fig. 1. Age and sex structure of the population for the United States: 2010, 2030, and 2050. (*From* Vincent GK, Velkoff VA. The next four decades, the older population in the United States: 2010 to 2050, Current Population Reports, P25-1138. Washington, DC: U.S. Census Bureau; 2010.)

mortality from cardiovascular-related diseases among young black men but not among older black men.[5]

MORTALITY

Reduced mortality at older ages is the leading cause of the increasingly greater life expectancy of the US population. A major shift has occurred in the past century regarding the leading causes of death for all age groups, including older adults: from infectious diseases and acute illnesses to chronic diseases and degenerative illnesses.

The leading causes of death in the population aged 65 years and older in 2010 were heart disease (24.2%), cancer (23.3%), chronic lower respiratory diseases (5.6%), cerebrovascular disease (5.2%), accidents (4.9%), and Alzheimer disease (3.4%) **(Fig. 2)**.[6] During the past 50 years, significant advances have occurred in both prevention and treatment of cardiac and cerebrovascular disease. Between 1981 and 2009, age-adjusted death rates for all causes of death among people aged 65 years and older declined by 25%. This decrease is largely attributed to a greater than 50% decrease in the mortality related to heart disease and stroke[7] in the 65 years and older age group. Cancer mortality rates increased in older men, however, with increases of 25% in men aged 75 to 84 years and 40% in men aged 85 years and older, mostly because of heavy cigarette smoking in older men at the end of the past century.[8] Concomitantly, death rates for chronic lower respiratory diseases increased by 57% between 1981 and 2009. Diabetes mortality rates similarly do not increase greatly with age because these patients disproportionately die at younger ages; however, the increasing incidence of obesity in the older population may lead to an increase in the incidence of diabetes.[9]

Alzheimer disease continues to increase as a cause of death in the older population, increasing 68% between 2000 and 2010, whereas deaths from other major diseases decreased; however, this is likely an underestimation, and the contribution of Alzheimer disease will likely continue to grow substantially.[10]

The mortality rate of accidents increases with advancing age, with 4 times as many deaths caused by other types of accidents, primarily falls, than from motor vehicle accidents.[11]

DISEASE STATUS
Health Care Use

With increasing age, the number of physician visits increases steadily. On average, persons aged 75 years and older have more than 7 visits per person per year. Acute

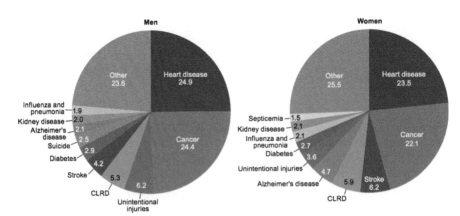

Fig. 2. Percent distribution of the 10 leading causes of death, by sex: United States, 2010 CLRD: chronic lower respiratory diseases. (*From* Heron M. Deaths: leading causes for 2010. National vital statistics reports, vol. 62. 6th edition. Hyattsville (MD): National Center for Health Statistics. 2013. p. 9. Available at: http://www.cdc.gov/nchs/data/nvsr62/nvsr62_06.pdf. Accessed April 29 2014.)

problems decrease steadily with increasing age, whereas the chronic problems become more prevalent, accounting for almost 60% of office visits in the age group older than 75 years.[10] Hospitalizations among the elderly population aged 65 years and older represent a significant portion of the annual expenditures on hospital care. Although the 65 years and older age group constituted only 13% of the US population in 2003,[1] they accounted for 36% of all hospitalizations, with more than 13.2 million hospital stays. The mean length of stay for patients aged 65 years and older was 1.7 days longer and the mean hospital charges 46% higher compared with the younger cohorts. Additionally, a larger proportion of hospitalizations among the elderly were through the emergency department.[12] Compared with the nonelderly, the proportion of in-hospital deaths for elderly patients was 5 times higher.[13] Hospital stays for the elderly resulted in hospital charges totaling nearly $329 billion, or 43.6% of the national hospital bill in 2003. The Medicare program is the third largest expenditure item for the federal government, and is projected to exceed Social Security by 2024.[14]

Causes of Hospitalization

The actual causes of hospitalization in persons aged 65 years and older (**Fig. 3**) are dominated by heart disease, including myocardial infarction, coronary artery disease, cardiac dysrhythmias, and congestive heart failure.[13] Pneumonia, stroke, and cancer are also common reasons for hospitalization and are associated with high mortality.

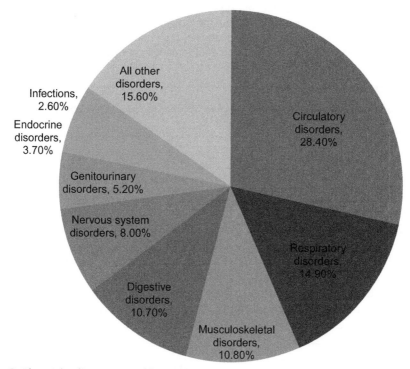

Fig. 3. The 10 leading causes of hospitalization in persons aged 65 years and older, first listed diagnosis. United States, 2004. (*Adapted from* Russo CA, Elixhauser A. Hospitalizations in the Elderly Population, 2003. Statistical Brief #6. May 2006. Rockville (MD): Agency for Healthcare Research and Quality; 2006. p. 8. Available at: http://www.hcup-us.ahrq.gov/reports/statbriefs/sb6.pdf. Accessed May 3, 2014.)

Other common reasons for admission include fractures, osteoarthritis, chronic bronchitis, and psychosis.

End of Life

Among older Americans, 49% of deaths occurred in hospitals in 1989, declining to 32% in 2009. The percent dying at home increased from 15% in 1989, to 24% in 2009. Use of hospice and the intensive care unit (ICU)/coronary care unit (CCU) is common in the last month of life. However, in the past decade, an increased use of hospice service and a decrease in intensive care stays at the end of life have been seen. In 2009, 43% of elderly decedents used hospice services in the last 30 days of life, representing an increase from 19% in 1999. Twenty-seven percent of elderly decedents used ICU/CCU in the last 30 days of life in 2009, compared with 22% in 1999. The length of hospice stay has also been increasing over the past decades. In 2009, 19% of hospice stays were more than 90 days, compared with 13% in 1999.[7]

COMORBIDITY
Chronic Conditions

In general, the risk of developing most diseases increases progressively with age. Thus, it is not surprising that the prevalence and severity of comorbidities, and the co-occurrence of multiple chronic conditions, are significantly higher in the older population. An estimated 2 of every 3 older Americans have multiple chronic conditions.[15] **Table 1** lists the most commonly reported chronic conditions in adults aged 65 years and older. Hypertension is the most common condition, reported by almost half of the older population, with nearly one-quarter of men and women reporting coronary heart disease. More than 8% of the older population reported a history of stroke.

Table 1 Most commonly reported chronic conditions per 100 persons aged 65 years and older in 2005		
Condition	Men	Women
Hypertension	44.6	51.1
Arthritis diagnosis	40.4	51.4
Chronic joint symptoms	39.7	47.7
Coronary heart disease	24.3	16.5
Cancer (any type)	23.2	17.5
Vision impairment	14.9	18.7
Diabetes	16.9	14.7
Sinusitis	11.5	16
Ulcers	13.1	10.4
Hearing impairment	14.8	8.4
Stroke	8.9	8.2
Emphysema	6.3	4.1
Chronic bronchitis	4.5	6.3
Kidney disorders	4.1	3.9
Liver disease	1.4	1.4

Data from Guralnik JM, Ferrucci L. Demography and epidemiology. In: Halter JB, Ouslander JG, Tinetti ME, et al, editors. Hazzard's geriatric medicine and gerontology. 6th edition. New York: McGraw-Hill; 2009. p. 9. Available at: http://accessmedicine.mhmedical.com.proxy.lib.umich.edu/content.aspx?bookid=371&Sectionid=41587608. Accessed May 10, 2014.

The prevalence rates of chronic conditions vary, however, according to race and ethnicity. In the subgroup of adults aged 70 years and older, non-Hispanic blacks have a 1.5-fold higher incidence of hypertension, with increased rates of stroke.[10]

Obesity

Obesity is a risk factor for many chronic conditions, including type 2 diabetes, hypertension, hyperlipidemia, stroke, heart disease, cancer (endometrial, colon, postmenopausal breast), and arthritis. Higher grades of obesity are associated with excess mortality, primarily from cardiovascular disease, diabetes, and certain cancers.[9,16–18] Between 1999 and 2008 the prevalence of obesity in men aged 60 years and older increased significantly from 33% to 40%, whereas the percentage of women who were obese declined from 39% to 35%.[19] During the same period, the prevalence of obesity among older non-Hispanic black men increased from 26% to 38%.[19]

Diabetes

The prevalence of diabetes among Americans older than 65 years varies from 22% to 33%.[20] Diabetes in older adults is associated with higher mortality, increased risk of hospitalization, and decreased functional status.[21] Older patients with diabetes experience higher rates of acute and chronic microvascular and cardiovascular complications of the disease. Of the obesity-related conditions, diabetes is most closely linked to obesity. Increasing rates of overweight and obesity in the older US population are strongly linked to the current epidemic of type 2 diabetes. With the aging of the US population, the Centers for Disease Control and Prevention projects that the prevalence of diabetes will double in the next 20 years.[22] Other projections suggest a 4.5-fold increase in the diagnosis of diabetes in adults older than 65 years between 2005 and 2055. In this period, minority groups will have the largest increases in the incidence of diabetes; the number is projected to increase 481% among Hispanics, 208% among blacks, and 113% among whites.[23]

Cancer

With the aging of the US population, a significant increase in the number of cancer diagnoses is projected. The US population is expected to increase 19% from 2010 to 2030, with a 67% increase in the cancer incidence anticipated for patients aged 65 years or older (from 1.0 to 1.6 million).[8] Prostate, lung, colon and rectum, and bladder cancers are the most common cancers that affect men, whereas breast, colon and rectum, lung, and uterine cancers are the leading cancers in women. With increasing age, the incidence of most of these cancers increases, but at the oldest ages, cancers such as prostate, breast, and lung begin to decrease in incidence.[24]

Dementia

The cause of most dementia is unknown, but the final stages are usually associated with a decline in cognitive ability, including memory and speech, and multiple other functions that are required for independent living. With a growth in the older population, the increasing prevalence of dementia will have a deep impact not only on the individuals and their families but also on the health care systems. In 2010, the estimated prevalence of dementia among Americans older than 70 years was 14.7%.[25]

Alzheimer disease is the most common form of dementia, accounting for 40.0% to 80.0% of these CNS illnesses.[26] In 2014, an estimated 5.2 million Americans were diagnosed with Alzheimer disease, including an estimated 5.0 million people aged 65 years and older.[27] With the increasing number of people in the United States falling into the elderly age group, the annual incidence of Alzheimer and other dementias is projected to double by 2050.[28] Alzheimer disease is one of the costliest chronic diseases to society because of substantial health care, long-term care, and hospice expenses. In 2014, total payments for all individuals with Alzheimer disease and other dementias are estimated to reach $214 billion, with Medicare and Medicaid covering approximately 70.0% of the total health-related expenditures for people with Alzheimer disease and other dementias.[25]

Disability

With increasing age, the prevalence of activities of daily living (ADL) disability increases rapidly, approaching 90% in persons aged 85 years and older.[29] In women and men aged 65 to 69 years, the prevalence of disabling immobility was 18.8% and 13.3%, respectively, and for women and men aged 90 to 95 years it was 83.3% and 63.4%, respectively.[30] More than half of adults aged 65 years and older report limitations in basic activities of daily living, such as dressing and bathing.[29] Chronic conditions, including acute events such as hip fracture and cerebrovascular disease and slowly progressive diseases such as arthritis and heart disease, are the major underlying causes of physical disability in the elderly[31]; additionally, the increasing incidence of obesity in the elderly continues to be a growing cause of disability.

Trauma

Traumatic injuries are important causes of morbidity and mortality in older adults, and older adults constitute a growing proportion of trauma patients in emergency departments. The increased population of older adults with active lifestyles has led to a dramatic increase in geriatric traumas. In 2008, adults in the United States aged 65 years and older accounted for more than 5.8 million emergency department visits for injuries, contributing to 30% of all visits by older adults and almost 14% of all injury-related emergency department visits.[32] Injuries sustained are more severe in older versus younger adults, and with the increased presence of comorbid disease and independent effects of age, this leads to increased morbidity and mortality in older patients.[33] Falls are the leading mechanism of injury and the leading cause of injury-related death in patients older than 65 years.[34] Falls accounted for 2.1 million emergency department visits among those aged 65 years and older in 2008; almost 10 times more common than motor vehicle accidents, the second leading cause of trauma in older adults.[11,35]

SUMMARY

The population in the United States is projected to grow older in the next several decades. Much of this aging is due to the baby boom generation moving into the ranks of the 65 years and older population. The aging of the population will have wide-ranging implications on the health care system. An understanding of the demographics of this special population and thoughtful planning is essential to prepare for the future.

REFERENCES

1. Vincent GK, Velkoff VA. The next four decades, the older population in the United States: 2010 to 2050, Current Population Reports, P25-1138. Washington, DC: U.S. Census Bureau; 2010.
2. Shrestha LB, Heisler EJ. The Changing Demographic Profile of the United States Available at: http://www.fas.org/sgp/crs/misc/RL32701.pdf. Accessed April 20, 2014.

3. Jacobsen LA, Kent M, Lee M, et al. America's aging population. Popul Bull 2011; 66(1). Available at: http://www.prb.org/pdf11/aging-in-america.pdf. Accessed April 15, 2014.
4. Arias E. United States life tables, 2006, Table A. Natl Vital Stat Rep 2010;58(21): 1–40.
5. Harper S, Lynch J, Burris S, et al. Trends in the black-white life expectancy gap in the United States, 1983-2003. JAMA 2007;297(11):1224–32.
6. Heron M. Deaths: leading causes for 2010. 6th edition. National vital statistics reports, vol. 62. Hyattsville (MD): National Center for Health Statistics; 2013. Available at: http://www.cdc.gov/nchs/data/nvsr/nvsr62/nvsr62_06.pdf. Accessed April 29. 2014.
7. Federal Interagency Forum on Aging-Related Statistics. Older Americans 2012: key indicators of well-being. Washington, DC: Federal Interagency Forum on Aging-Related Statistics; 2012. Available at: http://www.agingstats.gov/Main_Site/Data/2012_Documents/docs/EntireChartbook.pdf. Accessed April 19, 2014.
8. Smith BD, Smith GL, Hurria A, et al. Future of cancer incidence in the United States: burdens upon an aging, changing nation. J Clin Oncol 2009;27(17): 2758–65.
9. Must A, Spadano J, Coakley EH, et al. The disease burden associated with overweight and obesity. JAMA 1999;282(16):1523–9.
10. Guralnik JM, Ferrucci L. Demography and epidemiology. In: Halter JB, Ouslander JG, Tinetti ME, et al, editors. Hazzard's geriatric medicine and gerontology. 6th edition. New York: McGraw-Hill; 2009. Available at: http:// accessmedicine.mhmedical.com.proxy.lib.umich.edu/content.aspx?bookid=371& Sectionid=41587608. Accessed May 10, 2014.
11. Centers for Disease Control and Prevention. Web–based Injury Statistics Query and Reporting System (WISQARS). Available at: http://www.cdc.gov/injury/ wisqars/index.html. Accessed April 20, 2014.
12. Steiner C, Elixhauser A, Schnaier J. The healthcare cost and utilization project: an overview. Eff Clin Pract 2002;5(3):143–51.
13. Russo CA, Elixhauser A. Hospitalizations in the elderly population, 2003. Statistical Brief #6. May 2006. Rockville (MD): Agency for Healthcare Research and Quality; 2006. Available at: http://www.hcup-us.ahrq.gov/reports/statbriefs/sb6. pdf. Accessed May 3, 2014.
14. Centers for Medicare and Medicaid Services. 2013 Annual Report of the Boards of Trustees of the Federal Hospital Insurance and Federal Supplementary Medical Insurance Trust Funds. Washington (DC): U.S. Department of Health and Human Services; 2013. Available at: http://downloads.cms.gov/files/TR2013.pdf. Accessed April 29, 2014.
15. National Center for Health Statistics. Health, United States, 2010: With Special Feature on Death and Dying. Hyattsville (MD): National Center for Health Statistics; 2010. Available at: http://www.cdc.gov/nchs/data/hus/hus10.pdf. Accessed April 23, 2014.
16. U.S. Department of Health and Human Services. The Surgeon General's call to action to prevent and decrease overweight and obesity. Rockville (MD): U.S. Department of Health and Human Services, Public Health Service, Office of the Surgeon General; 2001. Available at: http://www.ncbi.nlm.nih.gov/books/ NBK44206/. Accessed April 20, 2014.
17. Moyer VA. Screening for and management of obesity in adults: U.S. Preventive Services Task Force recommendation statement. Ann Int Med 2012;157(5): 373–8.

18. U.S. Preventive Services Task Force. Screening for obesity in adults: recommendations and rationale. Ann Intern Med 2003;139(11):930–2.
19. Flegal KM, Carroll MD, Ogden CL, et al. Prevalence and trends in obesity among US adults, 1999-2008. JAMA 2010;303(3):235–41.
20. Kirkman MS, Briscoe VJ, Clark N, et al. Diabetes in older adults. Diabetes Care 2012;35(12):2650–64.
21. Brown AF, Mangione CM, Saliba D, et al. California Healthcare Foundation/American Geriatrics Society Panel on Improving Care for Elders with Diabetes. Guidelines for improving the care of the older person with diabetes mellitus. J Am Geriatr Soc 2003;51(5 Suppl Guidelines):S265–80.
22. Boyle JP, Thompson TJ, Gregg EW, et al. Projection of the year 2050 burden of diabetes in the US adult population: dynamic modeling of incidence, mortality, and prediabetes prevalence. Popul Health Metr 2010;8:29.
23. Narayan KM, Boyle JP, Geiss LS, et al. Impact of recent increase in incidence on future diabetes burden: U.S., 2005-2050. Diabetes Care 2006;29(9):2114–6.
24. Centers for Disease Control and Prevention. National Program of Cancer Registries (NPCR). Available at: http://apps.nccd.cdc.gov/uscs/. Accessed April 20, 2014.
25. Hurd MD, Martorell P, Delavande A, et al. Monetary costs of dementia in the United States. N Engl J Med 2013;368(14):1326–34.
26. Organisation for Economic Co-operation and Development. Health at a Glance 2011: OECD Indicators. OECD Publishing; 2011. Available at: http://dx.doi.org/10.1787/health_glance-2011-en. Accessed May 1, 2014.
27. Hebert LE, Weuve J, Scherr PA, et al. Alzheimer disease in the United States (2010-2050) estimated using the 2010 census. Neurology 2013;80(19):1778–83.
28. Hebert LE, Beckett LA, Scherr PA, et al. Annual incidence of Alzheimer disease in the United States projected to the years 2000 through 2050. Alzheimer Dis Assoc Disord 2001;15(4):169–73.
29. Motl RW, McAuley E. Physical activity, disability, and quality of life in older adults. Phys Med Rehabil Clin N Am 2010;21(2):299–308.
30. Leveille SG, Penninx BW, Melzer D, et al. Sex differences in the prevalence of mobility disability in old age: the dynamics of incidence, recovery, and mortality. J Gerontol B Psychol Sci Soc Sci 2000;55(1):S41–50.
31. Fried LP, Guralnik JM. Disability in older adults: evidence regarding significance, etiology, and risk. J Am Geriatr Soc 1997;45(1):92–100.
32. National Center for Health Statistics. National Hospital Ambulatory Medical Care Survey: 2008 Emergency Department Summary Tables. Available at: http://www.cdc.gov/nchs/data/ahcd/nhamcs_emergency/2008_ed_web_tables.pdf2008. Accessed May 1, 2014.
33. Hollis S, Lecky F, Yates DW, et al. The effect of pre-existing medical conditions and age on mortality after injury. J Trauma 2006;61(5):1255–60.
34. Bergen G, Chen LH, Warner M, et al. Injury in the United States: 2007 Chartbook. Hyattsville (MD): National Center for Health Statistics; 2008. Available at: http://www.cdc.gov/nchs/data/misc/injury2007.pdf. Accessed May 1, 2014.
35. Labib N, Nouh T, Winocour S, et al. Severely injured geriatric population: morbidity, mortality, and risk factors. J Trauma 2011;71(6):1908–14.

Health Care

Economic Impact of Caring for Geriatric Patients

Preston B. Rich, MD, MBA*, Sasha D. Adams, MD

KEYWORDS

- Health care expenditure • Gross domestic product • Health care economics
- Third party payer • Medicare

KEY POINTS

- Health care costs represent a larger percentage of the US gross domestic product (GDP) than those of any other developed nation in the Organization for Economic Co-operation and Development. Economists estimate a 4% to 7% per annum increase, which could approach 30% of GDP by 2035 if unchecked.
- Medicare (part A) payments exceed committed payroll tax revenue, and if they continue to increase at current rates, the Trust Fund assets will be depleted by 2017.
- The world's population is aging more rapidly than at any time in the past, in part because of prolongation of life expectancy; in the United States, the number of Americans older than 65 years will more than double in the next several decades.
- Although the elderly comprise only 13% of the US population, nearly half of all health care dollars spent are on the elderly.

INTRODUCTION: TRENDS IN US HEALTH CARE ECONOMY

With a gross domestic product (GDP) of $15 trillion, the US economy is the largest in the world, representing 20% of all global economic activity. US health care costs represent a larger percentage of this GDP than any other developed nation in the Organization for Economic Co-operation and Development (OECD) and result in the highest national per capita spending ($8233) in the world.[1] Historically, US health care expenditures have progressively outpaced growth in real income and have consistently exceeded GDP expansion by an average of 2.5% since 1975.[2,3] US health care spending increased from $27.1 billion (5.3% of GDP) in the pre-Medicare era of 1960 to $2.6 trillion in 2010 (17.6% of GDP).[1] Over the same period,

Financial Disclosure: Nothing to disclose.
Division of Acute Care Surgery, Department of Surgery, The University of North Carolina at Chapel Hill, 4008 Burnett Womack Building, Campus Box #7228, Chapel Hill, NC 27599-7228, USA
* Corresponding author.
E-mail address: prich@med.unc.edu

Surg Clin N Am 95 (2015) 11–21
http://dx.doi.org/10.1016/j.suc.2014.09.011
0039-6109/15/$ – see front matter © 2015 Elsevier Inc. All rights reserved.

surgical.theclinics.com

the percentage of health care costs paid for by the US government (federal and state) progressively increased, such that public sources account for nearly 50% of all payments.[3]

Economists project that health care costs will continue to increase at a rate of 4% to 7% per annum (forecasts are highly dependent on public policy and legislative action), a rate that if unabated will expand health care spending as a percentage of GDP to 30% by 2035 and will exceed 50% of all US economic transactions in aggregate by 2080. Federal financing of health care is already facing profound shortfalls, with Medicare Part A payments exceeding committed payroll tax revenue. If Medicare costs continue to increase at contemporary rates, the Trust Fund assets will be depleted by 2017. Given simple economics, it is evident that the increasing costs of health care may represent the single greatest threat to the economic security of the US population.

KEY DRIVERS OF HEALTH CARE SPENDING

There is increasing consensus that the disproportionate increase in health care costs is unsustainable and must be controlled given realistic expectations for associated growth in GDP. Although the major factors that contribute to cost acceleration can be reasonably well identified and agreed, there is more controversy regarding the relative magnitude and economic importance of the various components. The aging of the baby boomer generation is commonly believed to be a major driving force for the increase in overall health care expenditures. However, despite the increasing proportion of the elderly and the higher per capita spending incurred by this group, most economists attribute only about 3% of the cumulative increase in health care spending to this 1 driver.

Health care as a commodity is effectively a surrogate for the underlying associated values, which are the quality of health itself and the desire to maximize both individual and collective welfare. There is little doubt that in many cases, health care spending and resource allocation can be directly translated into the development of productive technological developments, the prolongation of life, the relief of suffering, and a measurable improvement in the quality of health. However, cost, quality, and well-being are not always directly related. From the perspective of economic efficiency and the appropriate allocation of scare resources, this nonlinear relationship necessitates the distribution of our scarce resources within the broader context of efficacy, cost-effectiveness, comparative analysis, and efficiency.

Technology

As the United States has transitioned from its manufacturing-based industrial revolution to an economy that is 80% service oriented, Americans have grown accustomed to rapid disruptive innovation and the development of advanced technological breakthroughs that fundamentally alter the structure and function of markets. In no sector is this phenomenon more evident than in health care. The development of new drugs, devices, services, procedures, and applications not only affects treatment paradigms but in many cases also expands possible treatments to new populations. Technological advances often outpace our ability to adequately study their effectiveness, and evidence-based strategies designed to rationally apply them are often replaced by their rapid and unsystematic adoption with unpredictable incorporation into medical practice. Although the potential exists for innovative technological advancements to decrease the cost of health care by reducing hospitalization or avoiding associated morbidity, most experts agree that most medical technological developments significantly increase the costs of health care.[4] Even when cost reductions are possible, technology expansion and application into broader populations have the net effect of increasing spending. Although measuring the direct financial impact of technology can be difficult, the cost contribution of technology on health care spending can be estimated as the cost residual that remains after accounting for more readily measurable drivers. Using this methodology, the Congressional Budget Office (CBO) estimates that approximately 50% of the growth in US health care costs can be attributed to technology, making it the single greatest contributor to health spending.[5] It is reasonable to predict that desirable technologies will continue to be developed in the future, perhaps at an even greater pace, further complicating our decisions regarding allocation of our limited resources.[2]

Insurance

Although health insurance was initially conceived as a mechanism to reduce the financial impact of catastrophic illness, its role has expanded in attempts to make all types of health care financially accessible and available to the population. As health care costs have continued to increase, the amount of out-of-pocket expenses paid by the end user has almost inversely decreased.[6,7] Although causality in this relationship is difficult to directly establish, a classic experiment conducted by the RAND Corporation from 1974 to 1982 provided strong evidence that reductions in coinsurance lead to more people using health services and more services used per person.[8] On the other hand, cost sharing reduced the use of both inappropriate and appropriate medical services. Although this effect had minimal consequences on the health status of most people enrolled in the study, for those who were poor and suffered chronic illnesses, the reduction in health use was harmful. The CBO concluded that between 5% and 20% of the increase in health costs can be attributed to the progressive expansion of more extensive health care coverage. One economist estimates that the insurance expansion represented by the institution of Medicare in 1965 may explain nearly half of the increase in health care spending that occurred between 1950 and 1990.[2,9]

Administrative and Overhead Costs

As medical care and its financial components become more complex, so must the infrastructure that sustains it. Although the administrative costs required to deliver health care can be difficult to accurately capture and gauge comprehensively, few would argue that the associated expenditures are increasing. Historical estimates attribute 3% to 10 % of increasing costs simply to increases in administrative and support functions in the sector. The CBO found that administrative costs increased approximately 7% year over year between the 1995 and 2005 fiscal years.

Malpractice Liability

The role of medical malpractice liability on escalating health costs relates both to the measurable impact of increasing insurance costs paid by providers and the less quantifiable but arguably more significant contribution of increased costs related to the practice of defensive medicine. Because malpractice premiums constitute only 1% to 2% of US health care expenditures, the projected 6% direct reduction in premiums that would likely result from tort reform would be expected to have only a modest impact on total expenditures.[10] This larger potential issue is also the most controversial: the notion that health care costs are driven dramatically higher by medical practice, which may overuse medical resources solely to reduce the chance of litigation. Several studies designed to address this issue have provided disparate results, and the relationship between malpractice liabilities and global health care costs remains in large part unanswered.[2]

Standard of Living

Because health and wellness are desired states of being, health care, as their market-based surrogate, is also a desired service. As personal income increases, one's ability to pay for a variety of health care services increases. Health care is a normal good, such that aggregate demand for it increases as income increases. Furthermore, because there are few substitutes available to replace it, health care shows significant price elasticity of its demand function. Consumers are fairly price insensitive, and this effect is further magnified by the relative disengagement of payment and services that occurs from the interposition of third-party intermediaries. A high per capita income in the United States is often cited as one of the key factors that contribute to our comparatively high health care costs. The true magnitude of this effect is a matter of debate, but economists have estimated the elasticity of US health care at approximately 0.2, meaning that for every 10% increase in real income, associated health expenditures can be anticipated to increase by 2%.[11]

CHRONIC DISEASE AND DISABILITY

In America, health care resources are not distributed equally among the population. To the contrary, the sickest 5% of the US population accounted for nearly half of all health spending in 2008 and 2009, and just 30% of the population account for nearly 90% of aggregate US health expenditures. The elderly are disproportionately represented among this top decile of spenders, comprising 13.2% of the population, but 42.9% of the heaviest consumers. Chronic diseases are more prevalent in the older population and their presence increases and maintains the increased costs of health care in this portion of the population.[12]

Chronic diseases, which affect older adults disproportionately, are the leading cause of death and disability in the United States, and modifiable conditions such as obesity and smoking are the most significant contributors.[13] In aggregate, the treatment of chronic diseases accounts fully for 75% of US health care costs.[12,14] In the United States, approximately 80% of individuals older than 65 years have at least 1 chronic condition, and 50% have at least 2.[14] The 10 most prevalent chronic disease diagnoses account for nearly one-third of national hospital charges. Of these diseases, the Agency for Healthcare Research and Quality identified 5 as sources of potentially preventable hospitalizations, given exposure to appropriate health modification strategies and preventive health measures (coronary artery disease, congestive heart failure, diabetes, chronic obstructive pulmonary disease, and asthma). The economic costs of chronic disease are cumulative; treating patients with 1 chronic condition (25% of the US population) costs twice as much as treating those without chronic disease. Treating patients who suffer from multiple comorbid conditions costs up to 7 times as much as does treating patients burdened by only 1 chronic condition.[13,15]

In addition to the increasing incidence of chronic disease, the aging process is associated with increasing disability secondary to sarcopenia or progressive loss of muscle mass. Approximately 45% of Americans older than 65 years are sarcopenic, with approximately 20% of the US population being functionally disabled.[16] When the prevalence of disability and the estimated increased cost for each individual are multiplied by the increasing number of older Americans, the economic burden of sarcopenia alone is estimated at $18.5 billion.[16]

The increase in obesity in the United States has been particularly problematic and costly to the US health care system. Obesity rates in the United States are now the highest in the world and have dramatically increased in all age groups over the last decade.[13,17] For adults, the obesity rate (body mass index [BMI], calculated as weight in kilograms divided by the square of height in meters, >30 kg/m^2) has tripled since 1960, and the incidence of morbid obesity (BMI >40 kg/m^2) has risen 6-fold. Because obesity raises the associated risks of major comorbidities, such as cancer, stroke, coronary artery disease, and diabetes, the impact of its effect on health is essentially magnified. In real terms, the relative cost of obesity was $1429 per year (42%) higher than caring for the nonobese population in 2006.[18] When combined with its prevalence, this high cost translated into $147 billion annually by 2008, or roughly 21% of US health spending: a cost that has now surpassed that associated with smoking.[19] As obesity rates continue to increase in the future, continued increases can be expected in associated chronic diseases and related health costs.

End-of-Life Care

Elderly patients undergoing elective or emergent surgical procedures experience significantly more 30-day serious morbidity and higher mortality when compared with younger patients.[20] Often, the perioperative care of the aging occurs in either a medical or surgical intensive care unit (ICU), and elderly patients account for approximately 50% of all ICU admissions, and nearly 60% of all ICU days.[21] Intensive care accounts for 20% to 30 % of overall hospital care costs in the United States, which was approximately $62 billion in 1992.[22] Of the patients treated in the top decile of expensive hospitalizations that included ICU care, 20% (2% of all hospitalizations requiring ICU care) died within 3 months.[22] The elderly account for more than 70% of all in-hospital deaths, according to the Healthcare Cost and Utilization Project (HCUP). The average hospital costs for a stay that ended in death was $23,000, which is 2.7 times higher than for a patient discharged alive.

HEALTH CARE PRICING

Some estimates attribute between 10% and 20% of increasing health costs to higher price trends prevalent in the health care sector. Although data patterns clearly support a progressive and significant increase in prices over time, an adequate analysis of their relationship to true cost is more challenging. Complicating these conclusions is lack of an effective and concurrent measure of comparative effectiveness and the impact of economic externalities. Because increases in technology tend to be associated with higher prices, it is unclear how much of a given price increase represents simple price inflation versus a marker of improved care, which may be associated with increased quality or even global reductions in total economic cost. It is plausible that some higher prices may generate cost reductions if the higher price yields even higher benefits from downstream associated effects, such as increased comparative effectiveness, superior diagnostic quality reducing unnecessary procedures, the avoidance of high-cost care such as hospital admissions or readmissions, or a subsequent decrease in the development or severity of chronic illnesses and conditions.

MARKET FAILURES IN THE HEALTH CARE SECTOR

The US health system has become increasingly complex, particularly from an economic perspective, as its overarching structure has progressively evolved from a fundamentally free-market system into a mixed system, which incorporates components of both free-market forces and the command attributes marked by government intervention that are common in many European health care systems. Although Americans typically regard the US health system as a free-market economy, various interventions, including the introduction of third-party payer systems, such as private health insurance and the development and expansion of government-sponsored programs like Medicare, Medicaid, and SCHIP (State Children's Health Insurance program), has generated many instances of what economists would refer to as market failures endemic in our system.

A market is a place, real or virtual, where sellers and buyers meet to execute transactions. Free markets show qualities of perfect competition, where each participant is considered a price taker, and no party possesses the unilateral power to influence the price of a product it either buys or sells. The laws of supply and demand determine prices, where a single price exists whereby the marginal benefit of obtaining 1 more unit exactly equals the marginal cost required to produce that 1 additional unit. This price, determined simultaneously by the market participants, is the only price that effectively clears the market. Such a perfect market shows Pareto efficiency, whereby no single market participant can benefit further by additional transactions without simultaneously disadvantaging another member.

Perfectly competitive markets have several key features that are each necessary to permit the ongoing efficiency of the marketplace. (1) An infinite number of market participants must be present and willing to both buy and produce a product at the market-clearing price. (2) There must be no barriers to exit or entry; any willing participant can freely enter or exit the market. (3) All buyers and sellers must possess perfect information about the prices, quality, and nature of the products represented in the market. (4) Zero transaction costs; buyers and sellers can incur no costs associated with the buying or selling of goods or services. (5) Firms show profit maximization, whereby they strive to produce and sell products at a price at which their marginal costs exactly equal their marginal benefit. (6) Products in the market must be homogenous, without variation across various suppliers. When 1 or more of these conditions is not met, market failure occurs, and the allocation of goods and services in a given marketplace is not economically efficient.

In practice, market failures occur commonly and are often associated with information asymmetries, noncompetitive markets, the existence of significant barriers to entry for new participants, and what are known as principal agent concerns problems, as occur with moral hazard, conflicts of interests, and misaligned financial incentives. Many would argue that the current system of health care delivery in the United States suffers from frequent and significant market failures that fundamentally alter its economics and contribute greatly to health disparities, inefficient allocation of scarce resources, and escalating costs that do not represent true market clearing prices and alter the nature of the relationship between supply and demand.

INFORMATION ASYMMETRY

An efficient and free market is highly dependent on the presence of perfect and inclusive information being readily available to both buyers and sellers about all marketable goods and services transacted on. Comprehensive information permits market participants to ascertain value, such that decisions about marginal cost and usefulness can result in an optimal and efficient clearing price. Perhaps in no situation is information asymmetry as apparent as in health care. The practice of medicine is highly specialized and difficult to understand, often with the superimposed potential for life-and-death outcomes, and aggravated by marked time pressure constraints, which preclude adequate information gathering. This extreme and almost universal asymmetry of information causes severe market failures, with the result often being inefficient resource allocation and price deflections.

PHYSICIANS AS AGENTS

Information asymmetry in health care produces an unusual relationship between market participants; patients rely on their providers to act as their advocate, or agent, with licensure and professional codes of conduct as quality control measures. However because physicians also serve as market suppliers with financial motives to provide goods and services, the potential for market failure is always present. This issue may result in supplier-induced demand, whereby providers allocate resources based on the potential for personal financial gain rather than to simply satisfy the health needs of a population.

BARRIERS TO ENTRY

In the 1960s, the American Medical Association (AMA) sought to restrict the supply of health care providers by introducing the requirement that physicians become licensed to practice medicine. Although this practice sought to ensure a basic standard of competence in health, it also restricted the supply of practitioners. In the early 1970s, a report from the Graduate Medical Education (GME) National Advisory Committee predicted an excess of physicians by 2000 if medical school and residency positions continued to increase. There was a voluntary moratorium on growth of medical schools, and a federal freeze on GME positions in 1997. These decisions were based on projections of US population growth that were underestimates of actual growth and did not take into account the increasing specialization of the physician workforce, both of which have led to an increasing shortage of physicians in the face of a rapidly aging population. The shortage has therefore led to reduced competition in the marketplace and an influx of physicians from alternative educational paths.[23]

MORAL HAZARD

The occurrence of illness is an unpredictable and costly event. Insurance markets have been developed in an attempt to mitigate this inhomogeneous risk and to financially prepare a priori for the uncertainty inherent in health and the human condition. By distributing risk among a population-based risk pool, the impact of individual unpredictability is diffused throughout a larger absorptive base. However, having insurance affects an individual's behavior through a phenomenon that economists call moral hazard. Because health care costs are paid by a third party, regardless of cost, insurance tends to induce an overconsumption of health care resources by the end user. Similarly, health care providers are subject to moral hazard as well; because prescribed treatments are known to be covered, insurance may induce the overallocation of health care. Both phenomena create market inefficiency and can result in the overuse of scare resources, which is a major driver of increasing health costs.

ADVERSE SELECTION

Insurance providers would ideally accurately price risk into individual insurance premiums to appropriately match cost with use. Because information is imperfect, risk assessment is necessarily incomplete. When premiums are set uniformly to reflect an average population-based aggregate risk, cost burden is unequal; the sickest users of health care pay less than their incurred costs, whereas the healthiest pay a disproportionately high cost for the goods and services they receive. In such a situation, the healthiest often forgo insurance and accept their lower perceived risk. This adverse selection results in only the sickest being insured at relatively underpriced premiums. Attempts to counteract this effect by pricing tiered premiums based on relative risk stratification results in very high health care costs borne by the greatest consumers of health care, effectively undermining the theoretic advantages of a distributed insurance pool.

IMPERFECT COMPETITION

A free market is dependent on the presence of large numbers (infinite in theory) of buyers and sellers, none having the individual power to influence supply, demand, or clearing prices. The last decade has witnessed the progressive consolidation of the health sector, with hospitals growing into health delivery systems and insurance carriers merging together in attempts to maximize efficiency through the leveraging of economies of both scale and scope. Consolidation can lead to the development of regional monopolies, which possess the capability of influencing market conditions, whereby individual entities set price, effectively becoming price makers rather than price takers. All of these trends have had the effect of reducing competition and altering the dynamic equilibria of supply and demand, generating inefficient allocation of resources and producing incentive for the escalation of health care prices.

EXTERNALITIES

In economics, externalities are unmeasured transaction spillover effects that represent either costs or benefits of a given market that are not reflected in the price of goods or services. Externalities reflect inefficiencies in a marketplace, and can either be positive or negative. Immunization is a classic example of a positive externality in health care. Most consumers purchase vaccinations for the tangible personal benefit of specific disease prevention. However, vaccination provides not only the consumer with benefit but also others in the population, who enjoy a reduced chance of infection, because the vaccinated can no longer spread the disease. This situation provides an important degree of social benefit (an externality), which is unmeasured on the individual transaction scale. Because the total benefit is a combination of individual benefit and the marginal social benefit (which is however unmeasured), society underestimates the true demand and therefore underallocates vaccinations. This effect in turn incurs a cost to society. Because of the tremendously complex matrix and inherent interrelatedness of both benefits and costs in health care, externalities are common sources of market failures.

LIFE EXPECTANCY AND LABOR FORCE

As the world enters the twenty-first century, most developed nations face pronounced structural alterations in their demographic profiles, marked by a progressive and sustained shift toward an older population. The world's population is aging more rapidly than at any time in our past, a global effect driven primarily by a relative reduction in fertility rate combined with a prolongation in life expectancy.[24] According to the United Nations Population Division, the number of individuals older than 65 years will outnumber those younger than 5 years for the first time in human history. The increases in life expectancy seen in OECD countries is profound; populations in developed nations can be shown to increase their life expectancy by 1 full day out of every 4. Globally, life expectancy has increased 3 months per year consistently since 1840, with no evidence of a plateau occurring.[25]

An important corollary of the relative expansion of the aging demographic is the simultaneous relative and absolute contraction of the employed labor force that contributes capital for societal consumption. As the leading edge of the expanded baby boomer cohort enters retirement age and produces an increased demand for goods and services, a reduced labor force is left behind to generate the required supply. In 1970, there were 5.3 workers for every postproduction retiree; currently, there are 4.6, and it is predicted that the ratio will decline to 2.6 workers per pensioner.[24,26] As the trend toward decreasing fertility and increasing life expectancy alters the demographic landscape for the foreseeable future, the imbalance between economic supply and demand from a population perspective will become even more extreme.[14]

Despite implementation of the comprehensive government-sponsored Medicare program in 1965, associated deductibles, copayments, and uncovered services generate a significant financial burden on the expanding aging cohort of Americans. As both demand and costs continue to increase, the individual economic impact of health care on American seniors will become increasingly significant. Assuming current insurance structure but projecting a systematic reduction in recent trends in cost escalation, the yearly out-of-pocket expense for Americans older than 65 years will more than double over the next several decades, whereas the median real income will increase more slowly.[27] As costs increase disproportionately to income, the percentage of real income required to maintain the current levels of health care service use will increase significantly from 10 % to 20 %. The percentage of senior Americans who spend more than one-fifth of their income on health care will increase to 45% by 2040.[27] Projections will be more dire for American seniors if cost containment is not achieved, and if employers eliminate current levels of retiree health benefits.

SUMMARY

National health care expenditures constitute a substantial and continuously expanding component of the US economy. In the context of a complex and rapidly evolving health delivery system, costs are increasing at an unsustainable rate and widespread market failures are exacerbating disparities in the efficient allocation of our scare resources. A meticulous analysis of health care spending patterns combined with an objective assessment of need can shed important light on how to best restrain increasing health care costs and simultaneously provide appropriate high-quality care.

Systematically identifying and characterizing the relatively small group of individuals who account for the largest percentage of US health spending may facilitate the introduction of targeted interventions into key areas in which their impact may be most profound. Changing demographics, an increasing incidence of chronic disease and progressive disability, rapid technological advances, and systemic market failures in the health care sector combine to drive exponential cost expansion, and a comprehensive multidisciplinary approach will become increasingly necessary to balance the delicate relationship between our constrained supply and increasing demand.

A consensus statement by the Council on Scientific Affairs of the AMA declared that "one of the most important tasks that the medical community faces is to prepare for the problems in caring for the elderly."[28] As the United States moves deeper into the twenty-first century, encumbered by increasing national deficits and a cumulative debt that may soon exceed GDP, it is clear that any plan to achieve sustainable quality care for our aging population will necessarily require seamless integration into an overarching strategy for our nation's entire health care system and the broader economy as a whole.

REFERENCES

1. OECD Health Data 2012. Available at: http://www.oecd.org. Accessed September 15, 2014.
2. Schieber SJ, et al. Social Security Advisory Board. The unsustainable cost of health care. 2009. Available at: http://www.ssab.gov. Accessed September 15, 2014.
3. National Health Expenditure Projections 2011-2021: Forecast Summary. Centers for Medicare and Medicaid Services. Available at: http://www.cms.gov. Accessed September 15, 2014.
4. Fuchs VR. Health care for the elderly: how much? Who will pay for it? Stanford Medical Review 1999;1(1).
5. Newhouse J. Medical care costs: how much welfare loss? J Econ Perspect 1992; 6(3):3–21.
6. Henry J. Kaiser Family Foundation. Trends in health care costs and spending. Menlo Park (CA): Henry J. Kaiser Family Foundation; 2009. Available at: http://www.kff.org.
7. Henry J. Kaiser Family Foundation. Health care costs: a primer. Key information on health care costs and their impact. Menlo Park (CA): Henry J. Kaiser Family Foundation; 2009. Available at: http://www.kff.org.
8. Brook RH, Ware JE, Rogers WH, et al. The effect of co-insurance on the health of adults. The Rand Corporation; 1984. Available at: http://www.rand.org/content/dam/rand/pubs/reports/2006/R3055.pdf.
9. Finkelstein A. The aggregate effects of health insurance: evidence from the introduction of Medicare. NBER Working Paper; 2005. Available at: http://www.nber.org/papers/w11619.
10. Paik M, Black BS, Hyman DA, et al. Will tort reform bend the cost curve? Evidence from Texas. J Empir Legal Studies 2012;9(2):173–216.
11. Liu S, Chollet D. Price and income elasticity of the demand for health insurance and health care services: a critical review of the literature. Mathematica Policy Research; 2006. Available at: http://www.mathematica-mpr.com/our-publications-and-findings/publications/price-and-income-elasticity-of-the-demand-for-health-insurance-and-health-care-services.
12. Cohen SB, Yu W. Agency for Healthcare Research and Quality (AHRQ) Statistical Brief. The concentration and persistence in the level of health expenditures over time: estimates for the US population, 2008-2009. 2012. Available at: http://meps.ahrq.gov/data_files/publications/st354/stat354.pdf.
13. Ehrlich E, Kofke-Egger H, Udow-Phillips M. Health care cost drivers: chronic disease, comorbidity, and health risk factors in the US and Michigan. Ann Arbor (MI): Center for Healthcare Research and Transformation; 2010. Available at: http://www.chrt.org.
14. Centers for Disease Control and Prevention (CDC). Public health and aging: trends in aging–United States and worldwide. MMWR Morb Mortal Wkly Rep 2003;52(6):101–6. Available at: http://www.cdc.gov.

15. Stanton MW, Rutherford MK. The high concentration of US health care expenditures. Rockville (MD): Agency for Healthcare Research and Quality (AHRQ); 2005.
16. Janssen I, Shepard DS, Katzmarzyk PT, et al. The healthcare costs of sarcopenia in the United States. J Am Geriatr Soc 2004;52:80–5.
17. Ogden CL, Carroll MD, Kit BK, et al. Prevalence of obesity in the United States, 2009-2010. NCHS Data Brief 2013;(131):1–8. Available at: http://www.cdc.gov.
18. Finkelstein EA, Trogdon JG, Cohen JW, et al. Annual medical spending attributable to obesity: payer- and service-specific estimates. Health Affairs 2009; 28(5):w822–31. Available at: http://www.cdc.gov.
19. Cawley J, Meyerhoefer C. The medical care costs of obesity: an instrumental variables approach. J Health Economics 2012;31(1):219–30.
20. Ingraham AM, Cohen ME, Raval MV. Variation in quality of care after emergency general surgery procedures in the elderly. J Am Coll Surg 2011;212:1039–48.
21. Menaker J, Scalea TM. Geriatric care in the surgical intensive care unit. Crit Care Med 2010;38(9):S452–9.
22. Yu W, Ash AS, Levinsky NG, et al. Intensive care unit use and mortality in the elderly. J Gen Intern Med 2000;15:97–102.
23. Sheldon GF, Ricketts TC, Charles A, et al. The global health workforce shortage: role of surgeons and other providers. Adv Surg 2008;42:63–85.
24. Lee R, Mason A, Cotlear A. Some economic consequences of global aging. HNP Discussion Paper. The World Bank; 2010. Available at: http://www-wds.world bank.org/external/default/WDSContentServer/WDSP/IB/2010/12/14/000333037_20101214003017/Rendered/PDF/584080WP0Box351lobal0Aging01public1.pdf. Topics: Health Nutrition and Population, Research: HNP Discussion Papers.
25. US Census Bureau 2012 Statistical Abstract. Available at: http://www.census.gov. Accessed September 15, 2014.
26. Coggan P. Falling short special report. People in rich countries are living longer. Without big reforms they will not be able to retire in comfort. The Economist 2011.
27. Johnson RW, Mommaerts C. Will health care costs bankrupt aging boomer? Washington, DC: The Urban Institute; 2010. Available at: http://www.urban.org.
28. Council on Scientific Affairs. American Medical Association white paper on elderly health. Arch Intern Med 1990;150(12):2459–72.

Effect of Aging on Cardiac Function Plus Monitoring and Support

R. Shayn Martin, MD[a],*, Jason P. Farrah, MD[b],
Michael C. Chang, MD[a]

KEYWORDS

- Elderly surgical patient ● Elderly cardiovascular anatomy
- Elderly cardiovascular physiology ● Cardiovascular monitoring
- Elderly cardiovascular resuscitation

KEY POINTS

- Elderly surgical patients are common and often require evaluation and support of the cardiovascular system.
- Aging significantly affects ventricular and vascular anatomy, resulting in altered cardiac functionality.
- Physiologic changes of aging include a blunted baroreflex and altered β-adrenergic responsiveness, resulting in a decreased dependence on chronotropy and an increased reliance on stroke volume in response to stress.
- Monitoring of the elderly cardiovascular system is valuable and can be achieved in several noninvasive and invasive methods.
- Management of shock in the elderly benefits from an understanding of the needs of the specific patient and a recognition of the risks and benefits of each cardiovascular medication.

INTRODUCTION

The world's population is aging and increasingly requiring medical and surgical therapy. As a consequence, growing populations of patients require care based on a specialized knowledge of the physiology of aging. Cardiovascular disease remains the most prevalent and influential comorbidity affecting outcomes in the elderly surgical patient. Although the elderly account for only 6% of the population, these individuals experience 30% of all myocardial infarctions (MIs) and 60% of all associated

[a] Department of Surgery, Wake Forest School of Medicine, Medical Center Boulevard, Winston-Salem, NC 27157, USA; [b] Department of Surgery, University of South Florida College of Medicine, 13220 USF Laurel Dr., 5th Floor, Tampa, FL 33612, USA
* Corresponding author.
E-mail address: romartin@wakehealth.edu

Surg Clin N Am 95 (2015) 23–35
http://dx.doi.org/10.1016/j.suc.2014.09.010
0039-6109/15/$ – see front matter © 2015 Elsevier Inc. All rights reserved.
surgical.theclinics.com

deaths.[1] The unique physiology of the aging cardiovascular system as well as the impact of these changes during the stress of surgery is presented in this article (**Table 1**). Further, the necessary response to these changes is discussed with attention to methods of monitoring and recommendations for providing supportive care.

EFFECT OF AGING ON THE RIGHT VENTRICLE

The right ventricle is connected in series to the left ventricle (LV) and is, therefore, obligated to pump the same stroke volume. As the cardiovascular system ages, this relationship is not always maintained and right heart flow may not always equal left heart flow. Both systolic and diastolic right ventricular function may be impaired with normal aging as demonstrated using echocardiographic techniques. Studies using M-mode echocardiography in combination with Doppler technology in healthy elderly volunteers have been able to explain impaired right ventricular systolic function. The tricuspid annular plane systolic excursion (TAPSE) estimates the longitudinal contractile properties of the right ventricle. These modalities demonstrate a significant reduction in TAPSE in otherwise healthy subjects as they age. Pulsed tissue–derived measurements of right ventricular systolic function have confirmed these findings, agreeing with findings of older studies demonstrating reduced systolic function on echocardiography. The mechanism for this reduction is believed to be secondary to a gradual age-related increase in pulmonary arterial vascular resistance, clinically evident by increased pulmonary artery systolic pressures.[2] This results in the exertion of more ventricular contractile effort into inefficient rotational motions, which has been observed using cine MRI.[3] Inefficient rotational motions and nonlongitudinal muscular movement contribute to the age-related decrease in right heart systolic function.

The aging process also affects right heart diastolic function. Diastolic functional properties can be characterized by determining right atrial pressure, tricuspid inflow velocity, myocardial early diastolic velocity (Ea), and atrial peak velocity (Aa).[4,5] Age is significantly correlated with progressive increases in Aa and decreases in Ea. Additionally, there is a negative relationship between the Ea to Aa ratio and increasing age, indicating less filling velocities in the ventricle despite higher atrial velocities.[4,5] In the same way that systolic functional decline is attributed to increasing stiffness of the pulmonary vasculature, diastolic functional changes are attributed to increased right heart afterload.[4]

Table 1 Summary of the effect of aging on the cardiovascular system	
Cardiovascular Element	**Alteration in the Elderly**
Right ventricle	Reduced systolic function Reduced diastolic function
Left ventricle	Left ventricular hypertrophy Dependence on atrial contribution Age-related impaired contractility and relaxation
Vascular structures	Increased arterial stiffness Systolic hypertension
Cardiac output	Preserved resting cardiac output Preserved ejection fraction
Changes in physiology	Blunted baroreceptor reflex Decreased adrenergic responsiveness
Response to stress	Decreased reliance on heart rate Increased cardiac output due to increased stroke volume

EFFECT OF AGING ON THE LEFT VENTRICLE

Years of ongoing stress on the heart results in changes in cardiac function related to increased workload. As aging blood vessels stiffen, leading to elevated systolic blood pressure, the LV changes in response. The heart is required to perform greater amounts of stroke work (stroke volume × blood pressure) in the presence of sustained elevations in systolic pressure, resulting in LV wall thickening in elderly patients.[6] LV hypertrophic remodeling is a recognized byproduct of the aging process although it is not known whether this is an adaptive response.[6]

Resting diastolic filling rates decline with age as evidenced by studies using M-mode echocardiography and gated blood pool scans. This decrease in early ventricular filling rate does not correlate with overall end-diastolic volume reduction suggesting that atrial contraction likely makes a significant contribution to ventricular filling in the elderly patient.[7] Decreases in cardiac output in the resting elderly patient were identified in previous studies although these studies did not differentiate patients with or without preexisting cardiac disease. Nevertheless, more recent studies have shown that resting cardiac output is preserved in the elderly patient without cardiac disease. Other indices of cardiac function (eg, ejection fraction [EF] and ejection velocity) were also preserved in these studies.[6,7] It seems that modest hypertrophic changes in the left ventricular wall are adaptive to preserve cardiac function. Other adaptations of the aging LV to maintain cardiac output include prolonged contraction, atrial enlargement, and increased contribution to LV filling.[6,7]

Cardiac MRI has recently challenged our understanding of left ventricular function in the elderly. Studies using cardiac MRI have investigated LV structure and function in large cohorts of ethnically diverse elderly individuals free of baseline cardiac disease.[8] This work demonstrated age-related decreases in LV mass in both genders as well as increased mass to volume ratios in the presence of decreases in LV end-diastolic volumes (LVEDVs). LV end-systolic volumes (LVESVs) were also decreased, resulting in a net decrease in stroke volumes that correlated with increased age. LVESVs were found to decrease less than LVEDVs, thus maintaining or modestly elevating EFs. Also identified was an age-related decrease in circumferential shortening during systole (age-related impaired contractility) and a decrease in circumferential lengthening in diastole (age-related impaired relaxation). Additionally, the increases in the mass to volume ratio of the LV were associated with an increased risk of subsequent cardiovascular events independent of age.[8]

EFFECT OF AGING ON VASCULAR STRUCTURES

Increasing arterial stiffness is the predominant change that occurs within the cardiovascular system in the setting of age. Even the healthy, elderly adult demonstrates age-associated increases in arterial stiffness that is proportionally greater in the diseased cardiovascular system. Potential energy released during the cardiac cycle stretches elastin fibers in the arteries and subsequently transmits this energy smoothly downstream to the muscular arterioles and capillary beds.[9] The aging process causes elastin to become depleted and replaced with increased amounts of nondistensible collagen and calcium.[10]

Age-related changes in the vascular structures result in a systolic hypertension syndrome that is characterized by an increase in systolic pressures with a lowering or maintenance of the diastolic pressure level resulting in a widened pulse pressure.[11] These changes in the walls of vascular structures predispose to nonlaminar and turbulent blood flow, which increases tensile and shear forces on the vessel wall resulting in progressive injury. To compensate for arterial stiffening, cardiac changes result in increased blood velocity to overcome the increased afterload of the stiffened central arterial tree.[12]

Vascular changes that occur due to aging result in compromised diastolic filling and, subsequently, the ability of elderly patients to tolerate the stress of injury or surgery. Central arterial elasticity decreases with age and is paralleled by increased pulse wave velocity occurring in the forward and backward (reflected) direction. Based on the intrinsic compliance of their vessels, young patients have pulse wave reflections occurring in diastole that augment coronary perfusion and ameliorate tensile shear forces of pulsatile blood flow.[12] Blood flow in less compliant vessels has enhanced shear due to turbulent flow and does not augment diastolic filling of coronary vessels that are already at risk due to atherosclerosis. A widened pulse pressure is the manifestation of stiffened central arteries due to a cardiac impulse transmitted downstream with greater force, causing reflected waves to return at end or peak systole.[12]

EFFECT OF AGING ON CARDIAC OUTPUT

Based on data generated from older technology such as M-mode echocardiography and gated blood pool scans, it was previously believed that, despite increases in vascular afterload, there was no significant change in cardiac output or pump function during the aging process. This maintenance of myocardial performance was thought to be due to increases in left ventricular thickness, a prolongation of contraction times, an enlargement of the atria, and an increase in the contribution of the atrium to left ventricular filling.[13] With the development of cardiac MRI has come an advanced understanding of the performance of the heart in the elderly. It is now recognized that, although older myocytes do increase in size, there is an overall myocyte depletion that is associated with increased collagen deposition and nonenzymatic cross-linking.[14] Although the older ventricle increases in overall mass, it does not increase in functional mass, as evidenced by increasing left ventricular mass to volume ratios and associated declines in LVEDV in relation to left ventricular mass. Further, although the resting EF is preserved, absolute stroke volume does not remain comparable.[8] Although both LVEDV and LVESV decrease with age, the decrease in LVEDV is proportionally greater than the decrease in LVESV, which leads to an overall age-related decline in resting stroke volume.[8] Age-related ventricular adaptation and decreased function over time is not unique to the LV. Right ventricular systolic and diastolic function similarly decline during the process of aging.[8] Although it was previously held that elderly patients could respond to surgical stress nearly as well as their younger counterparts due to a preservation of cardiac function at rest, it seems now that this is not true. The degree to which this affects the elderly surgical patient is poorly understood.[13]

EFFECT OF AGING ON THE BAROREFLEX RESPONSE

In the normally functioning cardiovascular system, the baroreflex serves as an efficient component of a complex feedback loop that maintains adequate cardiovascular function. The effect of aging on the baroreflex has been studied by relating pulse interval to changes in systolic blood pressure after phenylephrine injection. This work revealed a linear relationship between pulse interval and change in systolic blood pressure as well as a distinct decrease in the baroreceptor reflex sensitivity in the elderly.[15] Other investigators have found that an age-related decline in baroreflex sensitivity is independent of systolic blood pressure and systemic adrenergic levels.[16] Decreased baroreceptor reflex sensitivity was also demonstrated in a study of healthy volunteers examining cardiac response to angiotensin II (ANG II) infusions. The elderly, unlike younger patients, do not exhibit decreases in heart rate when blood pressure is increased via ANG II infusion.[17]

EFFECT OF AGING ON THE β-ADRENERGIC RESPONSE

The response of the cardiovascular system to surgical stress relies greatly on adrenergic stimulation. Unfortunately, one of the consequences of the normal aging process is a decreased responsiveness to β-adrenergic stimulation. Maximal heart rate (HRmax) decreases in the setting of aging and is responsible for decreases in aerobic work capacity. Decreases in HRmax are independent of gender, regular exercise, and other factors.[5,18] This attenuation of heart rate responsiveness contributes significantly to an age-related reduction in maximal cardiac output and, therefore, determines aerobic exercise capacity.[18]

The decrease in chronotropic responsiveness (HRmax) to exercise seen throughout the normal aging process remains poorly understood in terms of the exact mechanism.[18] The aging cardiovascular system demonstrates a decreased chronotropic and inotropic response to β-adrenergic stimulation, and this decreased responsiveness likely explains the observed decrease in HRmax.[18] However, studies of β-adrenergic responsiveness were performed using poorly matched, heterogeneous groups and have demonstrated inconsistent results. It has been found that differences in vagal tone do not seem to contribute to decreases in HRmax in normoxic conditions. Paradoxically, the aging cardiovascular system exhibits decreasing vagal tone when compared with younger counterparts, even in the setting of increased workloads during exercise.[19] One would expect this decreased vagal stimulation to enhance chronotropy but, nevertheless, HRmax remains decreased in the elderly.

Christou and Seals[18] have provided an understanding of age-related β-adrenergic responsiveness and decreases in HRmax. A cohort study involving young and elderly men examined the role of reduced intrinsic heart rate (HRint) and the effect of decreased β-adrenergic responsiveness on HRmax. HRmax was measured during treadmill exercise. HRint was measured at rest after complete ganglionic blockade, and β-adrenergic responsiveness was likewise measured at rest via exogenously administered isoproterenol after ganglionic blockade. The elderly were significantly more likely to have higher serum levels of norepinephrine at rest, lower HRmax, lower HRint, and decreased chronotropic responsiveness. Both decreased HRint and decreased β-adrenergic responsiveness were strongly related to decreased HRmax; however, HRint showed a higher degree of correlation. The study concluded that the decreased HRmax observed with aging is largely explained by a lower intrinsic heart rate that is present in healthy elderly adults.

Further work has attempted to elucidate the cause of lower levels of HRint in the elderly. One hypothesis is that decreases in HRint are a manifestation of occult sino-atrial node (SA node) dysfunction, possibly related to age-related myocardial fibrosis and collagen deposition.[20] However, SA node dysfunction is not always identified in the setting of myocardial remodeling and, instead, may indicate a molecular change in the pacemaker cells.[20] Studies have shown reductions in calcium channel proteins, which may lead to decreased sinus node depolarization reserve and, therefore, suppression of action potential formation and propagation.[21]

EFFECT OF SURGERY ON THE GERIATRIC CARDIOVASCULAR SYSTEM

Much of what we know about the response of the aging cardiovascular system to surgery has been elucidated from a body of work evaluating the impact of exercise. Surgery results in a substantial amount of physical and metabolic stress on the body due to blood loss, the inflammatory response, and the effects of anesthesia. The effects of stress vary greatly, depending on the age of the patient and the presence of associated comorbidities. Exercise provides a controlled stress state that allows some understanding of the effects of surgery on the elderly.

The normal response to exercise and presumably to surgical stress consists of an increase in cardiac output to meet the elevated metabolic needs of the body. Initially it was believed that the elderly demonstrated a depressed cardiac output response during exercise. Subsequent studies that excluded patients with coronary artery and myocardial disease showed a more appropriate increase in cardiac output, although the mechanism seems to be different than in the young.[7,22] Older patients cannot increase cardiac output with the typical increases in heart rate secondary to decreases in HRint and β-adrenergic responsiveness. The elderly optimize the Frank-Starling mechanism by increasing their end-diastolic volume and stroke volume during exercise, thereby increasing cardiac output without substantially increasing heart rate. Although the elderly are able to augment stroke volume during exercise, the increase in EF is less than that observed in younger counterparts secondary to a decreased ability to reduce end-systolic volume. This physiologic response is similar to that seen in young patients administered exogenous β-blockade and then stressed with increasing exercise loads. Finally, the elderly have increased plasma levels of epinephrine and norepinephrine during exercise loading, again reflecting the lack of β-adrenergic responsiveness.

Surgery and injury are frequently associated with hypovolemia secondary to blood loss and capillary leak commonly leading to cardiovascular compromise. Free water loss, chronic poor oral intake, pharmacologic vasodilation (home medications), and decreased plasma oncotic pressure (poor nutrition) also commonly lead to further intravascular volume depletion. Given the dependence on the Frank-Starling modulation of cardiac output instead of chronotropy, the elderly patient is particularly sensitive to preload reductions. Although Shannon and colleagues[23] showed that elderly patients mount a blood pressure increase and slight heart rate increase similar to younger patients during tilt tests, this response is negatively affected by hypovolemia. When the same test is performed after preload reduction with diuretics, elderly patients sustain a symptomatic decrease in blood pressure due to an inability to mount a tachycardic response in contrast to younger patients who exhibit an appropriate increase in both heart rate and blood pressure.

The literature evaluating the affects of exercise on the aging cardiovascular system has demonstrated the ability to maintain cardiac output in response to the stress of surgery.[7,22] The mechanism seems to depend on stroke volume by increasing end-diastolic volumes and contractility instead of augmentation of heart rate. Newer technology, including cardiac MRI and pulsed tissue Doppler echocardiography in 2D and 3D, has shown that, although elderly patients can mount a cardiac output response to stress, this is of lesser magnitude than in their younger counterparts due to decreased cardiac reserve.[7,24] Belzberg and colleagues[25] demonstrated these findings in a study of 625 trauma subjects who were monitored with a combination of transcutaneous perfusion devices and pulmonary artery catheters (PACs). Hemodynamic patterns for elderly (>65 years) and nonelderly (<65 years) subjects were analyzed and then stratified by survivors and nonsurvivors (elderly vs nonelderly survivors). Elderly trauma subjects had significantly lower cardiac index, heart rate, arterial oxy-hemoglobin saturations, and oxygen delivery. Although elderly survivors have significantly lower values of these parameters than young survivors, elderly and young nonsurvivors exhibit very similar hemodynamic and oxygen transport values. This study concluded that aggressive resuscitation titrated to hemodynamic and oxygen transport variables may improve outcomes and that the cardiac response to injury seen in elderly patients is much less robust than that of their younger counterparts.[25] It is clear that elderly patients generate increased cardiac performance in the face of the stress; however, the magnitude of this response is attenuated and less robust than that of younger counterparts. It is unknown whether this is due to normal age-related decline in cardiovascular function or to an increased prevalence of cardiovascular disease.

EFFECT OF COMORBIDITIES ON CARDIOVASCULAR FUNCTION: ATRIAL FIBRILLATION

Elderly patients rely heavily on prolonged contraction times and increased atrial contribution for adequate left ventricular filling. Atrial fibrillation (AF) is particularly problematic because atrial arrhythmias result in inconsistent and often inadequate ventricular filling due to limited contraction and decreased filling time. Age-related increases in left (and right) atrial size in older patients are a risk factor for the development of AF.[26] Additional age-related risk factors include inflammatory cytokines, local and systemic stress, altered calcium handling, and electrical remodeling on a chronic basis.[27] In the acute setting, pulsatile mechanical atrial stretch and inflammatory cytokines (from surgery, injury, or sepsis) contribute to arrhythmogenesis.[27] Numerous cytokines may contribute to development of AF, including IL-6, IL-8, and high-sensitivity C-reactive protein.[27] These same cytokines are present in high levels in the serum of injured patients and can be used to predict progression to multiple organ failure in the injured patient.[28] Surgical patients are exposed to other risk factors, including large-volume resuscitation, causing atrial stretch; increased endogenous catecholamine release; rapid fluid and electrolyte shifts; hypoxia; and hypercarbia.[29,30] Another common risk factor in the elderly is withdrawal from chronic β-blockade following surgical procedures.

AF significantly affects elderly surgical patients and frequently complicates the postoperative course. Chronic AF should be managed with the main goal being control of heart rate because this results in more optimal long-term outcomes.[31] Maintenance management of AF usually consists of β-blocker, calcium channel blocker, or antiarrhythmic medications such as amiodarone. These should be continued through the perioperative period as much as possible, although this can be challenging in the setting of hemodynamic compromise and limited gastrointestinal function. In the setting of significant surgery or severe injury, acute AF is common and results in prolonged hospital length of stay. There is no superior treatment regimen and therapy is usually tailored to meet the unique patient-care needs present at the time of diagnosis. Young trauma patients have been found to benefit from β-blockade because of the commonly high levels of catecholamines present at the time of injury.[32] For postoperative patients, β-blockade and calcium channel blockade are the most common and efficacious approaches in the presence of adequate perfusion. Patients with hemodynamic compromise at the time of AF onset may require synchronized cardioversion or the initiation of an antiarrhythmic such as amiodarone. Often, therapy for acute AF is only needed during the perioperative period and can be discontinued as the patient recovers, resulting in improved arrhythmogenicity. Nevertheless, AF should be diagnosed and managed expeditiously in the elderly because of greater expected reductions in cardiac output secondary to loss of atrial contraction and need for longer diastolic filling times.

EFFECT OF COMORBIDITIES ON CARDIOVASCULAR FUNCTION: ISCHEMIC HEART DISEASE

Surgical patients are at significant risk for acute myocardial ischemia given the associated endogenous catecholamine release, systemic inflammation, and increased myocardial oxygen demand. Additionally, hyperdynamic blood flow during resuscitation and its associated turbulent and nonlaminar blood flow increases shear forces in the vessel wall. This increased shear may cause the rupture of coronary atherosclerotic plaques and predispose to MI.[33] The risk of MI is compounded in the elderly in whom arterial pulse wave indices do not support diastolic filling of coronary vessels and arterial stiffening only exacerbates conditions of turbulent arterial blood flow. Elderly patients are also at greater risk due to preexisting coronary artery and intrinsic cardiac disease. Perioperative MI represents an important disease entity to address because it is associated with increased morbidity and mortality, especially in the aged.[34]

The elderly have the most risk of experiencing an MI after surgery; are most likely to suffer poor MI-related outcomes; and, subsequently, the most likely to benefit from intervention. Due to atypical symptomatology and presentation, MI is difficult to diagnose in critically ill elderly patients. A high index of suspicion and liberal use of diagnostic modalities such as electrocardiogram and serial troponin measurements are required to identify acute myocardial ischemia. Myocardial ischemia should be considered in the setting of unexplained vital sign decompensation after hemorrhage and hypovolemia are ruled out. Echocardiogram may be valuable to identify wall motion abnormalities in the face of nondiagnostic troponin elevation.[35] Cardiology consultation should be obtained liberally in the setting of acute coronary syndrome because the patient may be a candidate for reperfusion with coronary intervention.

EFFECT OF COMORBIDITIES ON CARDIOVASCULAR FUNCTION: HEART FAILURE WITH PRESERVED EJECTION FRACTION

Heart failure (HF) with preserved EF is defined as HF with an EF equal to or greater than 50%, and represents up to 40% of patients with heart failure.[36] This clinical condition is important because patients will seem normal when at rest and this resting EF is often erroneously used in these patients as a surrogate for achievable cardiac performance under stress. Several exercise studies of patients with HF with preserved EF demonstrated an inability to adequately increase LV systolic elastance. Further, these patients demonstrate lower peripheral resistance, increase heart rate, and reductions in ventricular-arterial coupling that result in an intolerance of submaximal and maximal exercise workloads.[36] Patients with HF express maladaptive inotropic, lusitropic, chronotropic, and vasodilator responses to the physical stress of exercise and are believed to have similar inadequate responses to the physical stress of surgery.

MONITORING THE AGING CARDIOVASCULAR SYSTEM

Due to the significant anatomic and physiologic limitations described above, the elderly cardiovascular system often requires multiple monitoring techniques to provide the necessary support during the perioperative period of time. The elderly do not have the same reserve as the young surgical patient and, therefore, require more exact maintenance of preload, contractility, and afterload to ensure adequate cardiac performance. The initial question that must be answered for any surgical patient should always be, "Is the patient in shock and underperfused?" The answer to this question is provided by clinical examination (mental status, peripheral pulse quality, skin temperature, urine output) as well as laboratory studies. Comorbidities are often present in the elderly and may mimic clinical findings such as dementia or delirium, chronic peripheral vascular disease, and chronic renal insufficiency. Laboratory findings such as lactic acid and base deficit remain valuable indicators of global hypoperfusion. At a minimum, an arterial catheter is required in any patient in shock, with marginal hemodynamics to provide continuous assessment of systolic and mean arterial blood pressure. More invasive monitoring techniques are often necessary to determine the intravascular volume status as well as cardiac and vascular abnormalities that may be present. It is important to recognize that the value of any monitoring technique highly depends on the ability to interpret the results of the device to appropriately make therapeutic decisions. The decision to implement a more advanced monitoring device should only occur when the clinician can no longer confidently describe the patient's intravascular volume status.

Modalities that provide the ability to monitor intravascular volume status as well as intrinsic cardiac function include arterial pulse waveform or indicator dilution analysis, PACs, and echocardiography. A central venous catheter measuring central venous pressure (CVP) provides the most basic assessment of intravascular volume status. Unfortunately, CVP is limited greatly by any factor that affects intrathoracic pressure such as mechanical ventilation. Therefore, CVP can be valuable when low, but a normal to elevated level does not rule out intravascular volume depletion. Systems that analyze arterial pulse waveforms attempt to determine the variability to stroke volume based on changes in the arterial waveform. Increased stroke volume variability can be used as an indicator of decreased intravascular volume that may benefit from volume expansion. Similarly, indicator dilution techniques use the peripheral arterial catheter by measuring the dilution of an injected substance from the time of venous injection to arterial sampling. This technique is capable of providing an indication of cardiac flow although this and arterial pulse waveform analysis methods depend on peripheral arterial blood flow and may be limited in the setting of peripheral arterial disease. A PAC provides pressure measurements from the pulmonary vasculature that better correlate with left heart filling, although it can still be affected by mechanical ventilation. Newer generation PACs provide calculated measurements of end-diastolic and end-systolic volumes, as well as blood flow and right heart EF that may be of greater assistance in optimizing intravascular volume status and cardiac performance. Despite studies challenging the value of PACs, when used correctly these devices continue to provide valuable information used to guide resuscitation especially in the elderly patient. More recently, bedside echocardiography used for resuscitative purposes has become more popular due to the ability to directly image the left heart. Both transthoracic and transesophageal methods are now available that allow the surgeon to visualize the left heart frequently without the challenges of obtaining formal echocardiography. These resuscitative echocardiographic techniques provide the ability to visualize and measure left heart filling as well as the associated EF. Repeat imaging after volume expansion or inotrope or vasopressor manipulation allows the clinician to immediately determine the impact of the recent interventions on improving cardiovascular function. The main challenge has been the education required to have adequate numbers of clinicians capable of obtaining the necessary images and the associated interpretations.

SUPPORT OF THE AGING CARDIOVASCULAR SYSTEM

The failing elderly cardiovascular system requires a careful determination of the cause of the inadequate perfusion. Most importantly, each patient should receive what he or she needs to correct the cardiovascular abnormality that is present. Unlike young patients, the elderly will often be intolerant to undercorrection or overcorrection, again due to the lack of reserve and the unique physiology that occurs with aging. Most surgical patients, whether young or old, require expansion of intravascular volume to optimize cardiac function. The elderly are more sensitive to hypovolemia; therefore, an early decision to institute invasive monitoring may be required to ensure the proper amount of volume expansion. Given that overresuscitation may be deleterious to the elderly surgical patient, this monitoring provides an opportunity to administer the appropriate amount of fluid. In the absence of portal hypertension physiology, crystalloid remains the most efficacious, safe, and inexpensive choice of fluid for volume expansion. Despite theoretic benefits, colloid has yet to demonstrate superior outcome results when compared with crystalloid alone.

When optimization of volume status fails to correct global hypoperfusion, correction of contractility and/or afterload with the initiation or modification of inotropes or vasopressors is required. The choice of agent remains a point of discussion throughout the surgical community. There are very little data supporting one agent compared with another, and the clinical scenario is likely more important than having standard medications of choice. Nevertheless, each of the agents has unique attributes that make them more or less appealing given the circumstances. Patients that have isolated contractility problems may benefit from dobutamine due to the specific myocardial stimulation that is provided via β_1-stimulation. Unfortunately, dobutamine can cause profound tachycardia that may not be tolerated in the elderly because of the significant increase in myocardial oxygen demand and the risk of precipitating AF. Although not as effective, milrinone provides enhanced myocardial contractile function without the effects on heart rate. Further, milrinone is appealing in the elderly due to its nonadrenergic mechanism of action given the presence of poor adrenergic responsiveness.

In the setting of decreased afterload, norepinephrine and vasopressin are commonly used to support hemodynamic function. Norepinephrine provides strong afterload augmentation via α-adrenergic stimulation while offering minimal β-stimulation on the heart. For this reason, norepinephrine is the most common vasopressor used in the setting of septic shock when there is a marked reduction in afterload. The result is an increase in blood pressure without affecting heart rate or contractility. Similarly, vasopressin is a noncatecholamine hormone that results in significant vasoconstriction and can improve blood pressure. Vasopressin does not function through adrenergic stimulation and, therefore, is appealing in the elderly patient who has blunted adrenergic responsiveness. Both norepinephrine and vasopressin benefit from increasing blood pressure without significant increases in heart rate, making them less arrhythmogenic. Nevertheless, it is important in the elderly, who have limited contractile reserve, to avoid implementing unopposed afterload augmentation that might result in myocardial decompensation and decreased cardiac performance.

When monitoring of the cardiovascular system reveals findings consistent with reduced contractility and afterload, epinephrine may be a valuable agent to provide support. Epinephrine stimulates both α-adrenergic and β-adrenergic receptors, resulting in enhanced contractility and vasoconstriction. The result is increased cardiac output and blood pressure, as well as improved coronary blood flow. With that said, tachycardia is common, resulting in increased myocardial oxygen demand and a greater likelihood of AF. Nevertheless, epinephrine is a valuable agent to use but should be selected carefully and the results monitored closely.

SUMMARY

The elderly surgical patient presents challenges related to anatomic and physiologic changes as well as preexisting conditions. Altered cardiovascular function is common in the elderly surgical patient, resulting in an inability to adequately perfuse the organs of the body. The elderly cardiovascular system exhibits a blunted response to adrenergic stimulation due to reductions in intrinsic heart rate and β-adrenergic responsiveness. The ability to increase cardiac output during surgery relies more on increased ventricular filling and stroke volume than on increases in heart rate and EF. The elderly also demonstrate decreases in baroreceptor reflexes that make them more sensitive to hypovolemia and hemorrhage. Atrial dysrhythmias are common and must be rapidly diagnosed and treated due to a reliance on atrial contributions for adequate ventricular filling and cardiac output. Monitoring of cardiovascular function may be more beneficial than in the young due to the importance of achieving optimal volume status. When inotrope or vasopressor agents are necessary, careful selection based on the specific needs of the patient is important given the unique risks and benefits of each medication. Frequent reassessment after initiating or modifying cardiovascular medications is required to ensure achieving improved perfusion and to monitor for untoward complications.

REFERENCES

1. Crispell KA. Common cardiovascular issues encountered in geriatric critical care. Crit Care Clin 2003;19(4):677–91.
2. Haddad F, Hunt SA, Rosenthal DN, et al. Right ventricular function in cardiovascular disease, part I: anatomy, physiology, aging, and functional assessment of the right ventricle. Circulation 2008;117(11):1436–48.
3. Sandstede J, Lipke C, Beer M, et al. Age- and gender-specific differences in left and right ventricular cardiac function and mass determined by cine magnetic resonance imaging. Eur Radiol 2000;10(3):438–42.
4. Innelli P, Esposito R, Olibet M, et al. The impact of aging on right ventricular longitudinal function in healthy subjects: a pulsed tissue Doppler study. Eur J Echocardiogr 2009;10(4):491–8.
5. Lindqvist P, Waldenstrom A, Henein M, et al. Regional and global right ventricular function in healthy individuals aged 20-90 years: a pulsed Doppler tissue imaging study: Umea General Population Heart Study. Echocardiography 2005;22(4):305–14.
6. Lakatta EG. Do hypertension and aging have a similar effect on the myocardium? Circulation 1987;75(1 Pt 2):I69–77.
7. Rodeheffer RJ, Gerstenblith G, Becker LC, et al. Exercise cardiac output is maintained with advancing age in healthy human subjects: cardiac dilatation and increased stroke volume compensate for a diminished heart rate. Circulation 1984;69(2):203–13.
8. Cheng S, Fernandes VR, Bluemke DA, et al. Age-related left ventricular remodeling and associated risk for cardiovascular outcomes: the Multi-Ethnic Study of Atherosclerosis. Circ Cardiovasc Imaging 2009;2(3):191–8.
9. O'Rourke M. Mechanical principles in arterial disease. Hypertension 1995;26(1):2–9.
10. Greenwald SE. Ageing of the conduit arteries. J Pathol 2007;211(2):157–72.
11. Izzo JL Jr. Arterial stiffness and the systolic hypertension syndrome. Curr Opin Cardiol 2004;19(4):341–52.
12. Nichols WW, Edwards DG. Arterial elastance and wave reflection augmentation of systolic blood pressure: deleterious effects and implications for therapy. J Cardiovasc Pharmacol Ther 2001;6(1):5–21.
13. Duggan J, Kilfeather S, O'Brien E, et al. Effects of aging and hypertension on plasma angiotensin II and platelet angiotensin II receptor density. Am J Hypertens 1992;5(10):687–93.

14. Olivetti G, Melissari M, Capasso JM, et al. Cardiomyopathy of the aging human heart. Myocyte loss and reactive cellular hypertrophy. Circ Res 1991;68(6): 1560–8.
15. Gribben B, Pickering TG, Sleight P, et al. Effect of age and high blood pressure on baroreflex sensitivity in man. Circ Res 1971;29:424–31.
16. Shimada K, Kitazumi T, Sadakane N, et al. Age-related changes of baroreflex function, plasma norepinephrine, and blood pressure. Hypertension 1985;7(1):113–7.
17. Duggan J, Nussberger J, Kilfeather S, et al. Aging and human hormonal and pressor responsiveness to angiotensin II infusion with simultaneous measurement of exogenous and endogenous angiotensin II. Am J Hypertens 1993; 6(8):641–7.
18. Christou DD, Seals DR. Decreased maximal heart rate with aging is related to reduced {beta}-adrenergic responsiveness but is largely explained by a reduction in intrinsic heart rate. J Appl Physiol (1985) 2008;105(1):24–9.
19. Ford GA, James OF. Effect of 'autonomic blockade' on cardiac beta-adrenergic chronotropic responsiveness in healthy young, healthy elderly and endurance-trained elderly subjects. Clin Sci (Lond) 1994;87(3):297–302.
20. Kistler PM, Sanders P, Fynn SP, et al. Electrophysiologic and electroanatomic changes in the human atrium associated with age. J Am Coll Cardiol 2004; 44(1):109–16.
21. Jones SA, Boyett MR, Lancaster MK. Declining into failure: the age-dependent loss of the L-type calcium channel within the sinoatrial node. Circulation 2007; 115(10):1183–90.
22. Port S, Cobb FR, Coleman RE, et al. Effect of age on the response of the left ventricular ejection fraction to exercise. N Engl J Med 1980;303(20):1133–7.
23. Shannon RP, Wei JY, Rosa RM, et al. The effect of age and sodium depletion on cardiovascular response to orthostasis. Hypertension 1986;8(5):438–43.
24. Innelli P, Sanchez R, Marra F, et al. The impact of aging on left ventricular longitudinal function in healthy subjects: a pulsed tissue Doppler study. Eur J Echocardiogr 2008;9(2):241–9.
25. Belzberg H, Wo CC, Demetriades D, et al. Effects of age and obesity on hemodynamics, tissue oxygenation, and outcome after trauma. J Trauma 2007;62(5): 1192–200.
26. Lakatta EG, Levy D. Arterial and cardiac aging: major shareholders in cardiovascular disease enterprises: part II: the aging heart in health: links to heart disease. Circulation 2003;107(2):346–54.
27. Hadi HA, Alsheikh-Ali AA, Mahmeed WA, et al. Inflammatory cytokines and atrial fibrillation: current and prospective views. J Inflamm Res 2010;3:75–97.
28. Frink M, van GM, Kobbe P, et al. IL-6 predicts organ dysfunction and mortality in patients with multiple injuries. Scand J Trauma Resusc Emerg Med 2009;17:49.
29. Solti F, Vecsey T, Kekesi V. Effect of atrial dilatation on the tendency of atrial arrhythmias. Acta Physiol Hung 1989;74(1):49–55.
30. Amar D, Zhang H, Leung DH, et al. Older age is the strongest predictor of postoperative atrial fibrillation. Anesthesiology 2002;96(2):352–6.
31. The Atrial Fibrillation Follow-up Investigation of Rhythm Management (AFFIRM) Investigators. A comparison of rate control and rhythm control in patients with atrial fibrillation. N Engl J Med 2002;347:1825–33.
32. Hadjizacharia P, O'Keeffe T, Brown CVR, et al. Incidence, risk factors, and outcomes for atrial arrhythmias in trauma patients. Am Surg 2011;77(5):634–9.
33. Moosikasuwan JB, Thomas JM, Buchman TG. Myocardial infarction as a complication of injury. J Am Coll Surg 2000;190(6):665–70.

34. Perdue PW, Watts DD, Kaufmann CR, et al. Differences in mortality between elderly and younger adult trauma patients: geriatric status increases risk of delayed death. J Trauma 1998;45(4):805–10.

35. Alcalai R, Planer D, Culhaoglu A, et al. Acute coronary syndrome vs nonspecific troponin elevation: clinical predictors and survival analysis. Arch Intern Med 2007;167(3):276–81.

36. Borlaug BA, Olson TP, Lam CS, et al. Global cardiovascular reserve dysfunction in heart failure with preserved ejection fraction. J Am Coll Cardiol 2010;56(11): 845–54.

Effect of Aging on the Vascular System Plus Monitoring and Support

Ed Villella, MD[a],*, Jae S. Cho, MD[b]

KEYWORDS

- Atherosclerosis • Endothelial progenitor cells • Nitric oxide • Arterial stiffness
- Oxidative stress • Aging

KEY POINTS

- Cardiovascular disease has become the most common cause of death worldwide.
- Many known factors increase this risk, including diabetes, smoking, hypertension, renal disease, and sedentary lifestyle.
- New studies have shown that the declining function of the arterial endothelium with age is an independent risk factor for the development of vascular disease in otherwise healthy adults.
- Strategies aimed to improve the overall integrity of the endothelium may reduce arterial stiffness and delay atherosclerosis formation.
- Optimizing endothelial function may improve cardiovascular health in an aging population.

INTRODUCTION

Cardiovascular diseases have become the most common cause of morbidity and mortality in the world today. Cardiovascular disease accounts for almost half of the deaths for people older than 65 and has an enormous impact on the health care system for treatment of vascular disease and its associated complications.[1] There are many known modifiable risk factors that lead to decline in vascular function; however, the most common nonmodifiable cause is aging. In otherwise healthy adults, aging has been found to be an independent risk factor for the health and function of the vascular system. There has been increasing investigation in this area because there is an expected rise in the elderly population over the next several decades. With advances in health care, it is expected that the number of people in the world

[a] Loyola University Medical Center, 2160 South 1st Avenue, EMS Building 110, Room 3210, Maywood, IL 60153, USA; [b] Vascular Surgery & Endovascular Therapy, Surgery and Cardiothoracic Surgery, Stritch School of Medicine, Loyola University Chicago, 2160 South First Avenue, EMS Building 110, Room 3215, Maywood, IL 60153, USA
* Corresponding author.
E-mail address: villella1224@yahoo.com

Surg Clin N Am 95 (2015) 37–51
http://dx.doi.org/10.1016/j.suc.2014.09.007
0039-6109/15/$ – see front matter © 2015 Elsevier Inc. All rights reserved.

older than 60 will more than double in the next 40 years and will account for more than 20% of the total population. As a result, we can expect to have an increasing number of vascular-related health issues for years to come.

It is well known that arteries become stiffer and less compliant with age.[2] This is attributed to repeated strain from pulsatile waves that lead to increased collagen deposition and a loss of elastin.[3] Other factors accelerate this process, such as hypertension, smoking, and renal disease. More recently, there has been growing investigation into the biochemical changes of the arterial endothelium that are hypothesized to be contributing to this process in patients who do not exhibit other risk factors. These studies have looked at nitric oxide (NO), oxidative stress leading to reactive oxygen species (ROS), telomere shortening, and endothelial progenitor cells (EPCs) to further define the main pathogenesis of arterial aging. Targeting these biochemical pathways has given rise to alternative treatment strategies that are directed toward improving the health and function of the endothelium at the cellular level in an attempt to slow the aging process of the arteries.

BASIC ANATOMY AND PHYSIOLOGY

The artery is composed of 3 layers: the tunica intima, tunica media, and the adventitia (**Fig. 1**). The tunica media is located between the intima and adventitia and contains structural components, such as smooth muscle cells, collagen, and elastin.[4] The adventitia is the outermost layer, and tends to be more prominent in the muscular arteries. This layer contains the vaso vasorum, which is the blood supply to the artery, and has direct communication with the surrounding tissues. The media is the stabilizing layer of the artery and provides the framework on which a vessel vasoconstricts and vasodilates. The intima is the innermost layer of the artery and is lined by the endothelium. It is in this endothelial layer that there is growing interest in investigating its role in the aging process of the artery.

The endothelium contains endothelial cells that participate in cell signaling to initiate muscular contraction or dilation, allow migration of molecules and ion exchange, and regulate the formation and dissolution of clot of an injured arterial

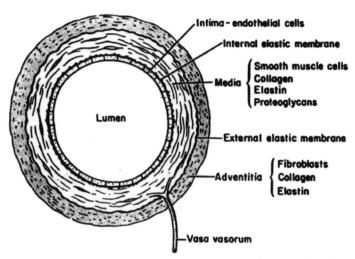

Fig. 1. Schematic of the layers of the arterial wall. (*Courtesy of* Institute for Advanced Medical Education. Available at: https://iame.com; used with permission.)

wall. NO is an important signaling molecule that is stimulated in response to leuko-cyte invasion or mechanical wall stress. Its precursor is from the amino acid L-argi-nine and is produced via an enzymatic reaction with nitric oxide synthase (NOS) and its cofactor tetrahydrobiopterin (BH_4). The main functions of NO include vasodilation, and inhibition of platelet adhesion and aggregation; it also contains anti-inflammatory properties.[3,5]

Another important molecule in the endothelium is the EPC. EPCs are derived from bone marrow or mononuclear cells and have various functions.[6] It is widely accepted that endothelial injury is the inciting event for which atherosclerosis is initiated and EPCs help to maintain the endothelium by not only acting as a repair mechanism, but also by differentiating into healthy endothelial cells that will restore tissue integrity.[7]

EFFECTS OF AGING ON ARTERIAL STRUCTURE AND FUNCTION
Structural Changes

The impact of aging on blood vessel structure and function is profound. Structural changes in large arteries include elongation and dilatation.

The arterial wall thickens due to changes in the intima and media.[8] Although no endothelial lesions are noted in healthy elderly individuals, the endothelial cells may be irregular in shape and have increased height. Migration and proliferation of vascular smooth cells may occur with infiltration in the subendothelial space. Increased depo-sition of collagen, elastin fragmentation, and proteoglycans by leukocytes and macro-phages also is noted.

Repeated mechanical stress from the pulsatile blood flow exerted on the aorta and arteries over a long time causes collagen deposition and a loss of elastin in the arterial wall, resulting in arterial stiffness with age.[9,10] These effects also are seen in more peripheral arteries, which are a result of an overall amplification of antegrade pulsatile force that is propagated downstream. Other factors involved with inflammation and atherosclerosis, such as cellular adhesion molecules, matrix metalloproteases, trans-forming growth factor-β, and proinflammatory cytokines, also are found in the aging intima.[11] **Table 1** details the changes that occur in the arterial wall with aging.

Functional Changes

The primary functional change that occurs with aging of large arteries is decreased compliance in the aorta and the larger arteries.[12] The resulting large-vessel stiffness greatly contributes to pathophysiology of hypertension and other cardiovascular diseases in older individuals.[13,14] At the level of small arteries and arterioles, the systemic vascular resistance increases with aging due to impairment of endothelial function, including altered responsiveness of the endothelium to the stimuli that regu-late the vascular tone, resulting in vasospasm and thrombosis of blood vessels.[15] Vascular endothelium also regulates vessel wall permeability, vascular tone, structure and blood flow, and facilitates anticoagulant and fibrinolytic activities. The main vaso-active factors released by endothelial cells are NO and cyclooxygenase (COX)-derived eicosanoids.

NO is derived from L-arginine and functions as a principal molecule in the regulation of vascular homeostasis. NO regulates larger artery compliance[16]; mediates the vaso-dilatory effects of substance P, bradykinin, and acetylcholine[17,18]; inhibits leukocyte adhesion; and has antithrombotic and antiapoptotic properties. Its production is regulated by 3 NOS isoforms: endothelial (eNOS), neuronal (nNOS), and inducible (iNOS). The eNOS and nNOS isoforms are expressed constitutively in vessels and

Table 1
Changes that occur to the arterial wall as a result of natural aging

Arterial wall thickness (intima-media)	Increase
Subendothelial collagen	Increase
Subendothelial elastin	Decrease
Elastin fragmentation	Increase
Proteoglycans	Increase
MMP activity	Increase
Intimal migration/proliferation of VSMCs	Increase
Arterial distensibility	Decrease
Pulse wave velocity	Increase
Total peripheral resistance	Increase
Endothelial permeability	Increase
Endothelial nitric oxide release	Decrease
Inflammatory markers/mediators	Increase
SOD activity	Decrease
Beta-adrenergic–mediated vasodilation	Decrease

Abbreviations: MMP, matrix metalloproteinases; SOD, superoxide dismutase; VSMC, vascular smooth muscle cells.

neurons,[19,20] whereas iNOS is expressed by vascular cells in response to external stimuli, such as chemokines and invading microorganisms.[21] NO generated by nNOS and iNOS is classically described as a neurotransmitter and a reactive molecule involved in bacterial killing, respectively.

Several studies in human and animal models have shown that endothelium-dependent vasodilatation, a marker of endothelial function, progressively declines with age.[22–28] Vascular aging is accompanied by reduced eNOS expression/activity or augmented breakdown of NO by ROS. The homeostasis between production and availability of NO is maintained by the normal activity of eNOS, whereas an excessive amount of NO production by upregulation of iNOS contributes to vascular dysfunction. In senescent endothelial cells, upregulation of iNOS may be associated with nuclear factor-κB–induced vascular inflammation, producing high levels of NO. When NO reacts with cysteine residues of arginase, it increases arginase activity and L-arginine consumption. NO reacts with the superoxide anion, generated by uncoupled eNOS, and produces the reactive nitrogen species peroxynitrite, which increases vasoconstrictor tone in senescent arteries.

In addition, aging endothelial cells phenotype shifts toward an inflammatory state, with upregulation of adhesion molecules, cytokines, and chemokines.[29] This phenotype favors platelet aggregation and inflammatory cell adhesion, which predisposes thrombosis and atherosclerosis. The expression of proinflammatory enzymes, such as COX-2 and iNOS, is induced by aging-associated endothelial dysfunction.[29] COX-2–derived lipid mediators can contribute to enhanced reactivity to vasoconstrictors.[30,31]

Decreased Bioavailability of Nitric Oxide

The decreased bioavailability of NO with age is thought to be a leading cause of the increased inflammatory and atherogenesis of the aging artery. There are many factors that lead to the depletion of NO over time (**Fig. 2**).

- eNOS is an enzyme released from the endothelium that catalyzes the formation of NO from L-arginine.[32-34]
- Decreased concentrations of L-arginine due to nutritional deficiencies lower NO production.[35]
- Increased enzymatic degradation of L-arginine by the enzyme arginase degrades L-arginine and decreases the availability of the substrate that forms NO.[33]
- Asymmetric dimethylarginine (ADMA) is an endogenous L-arginine analog that competitively binds to the NOS active site and ultimately impedes the formation of NO.[32]
- ROS decrease the bioavailability of NO by causing uncoupling of eNOS and reducing L-arginine and BH_4.[3]
- Downregulation of antioxidants with age allow for the proliferation of ROS.
- There is a reduction of cofactor BH_4, which is found on NOS and is necessary for the enzymatic production of NO from its substrate.[33] The availability of BH_4 is negatively impacted in the presence of ROS.

Altered Responsiveness to Stimuli

Aging vasculature is associated with decreased responses to various stimuli. The principal mediators of vasoconstriction in arterioles are the catecholamine α_1-adrenergic system, the endothelin-1/endothelin receptor system, and the renin-angiotensin system. They vary in their onset of action and duration of effect. The alpha$_1$-adrenergic receptor system is the fastest in onset but shortest in duration, whereas the endothelin receptor system is the slowest in onset but the longest in duration of action. It has

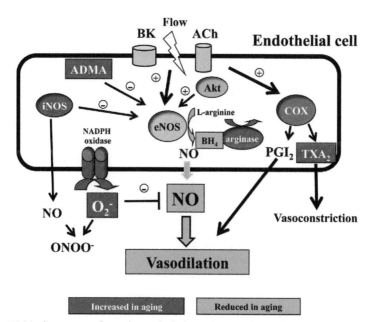

Fig. 2. eNOS is the enzyme from the endothelium that catalyzes the production of NO from L-arginine. BH_4 is a cofactor necessary for the catalytic reaction. Arginase breaks down L-arginine and decreases the concentration of the substrate for NO. ADMA is a competitive analog to L-arginine. A by-product of iNOS production of NO is NADPH oxidase, which leads to ROS formation. (*From* El Assar M, Angulo J, Vallejo S, et al. Mechanisms involved in the aging-induced vascular dysfunction. Front Physiol 2012;3(132):3; with permission.)

been shown that the responsiveness of arterioles to the catecholamine α_1-adrenergic receptor decreases with aging; intra-arterial noradrenaline infusion results in more reduced vasoconstriction in older adults than in younger cohorts.[36,37]

The major mediator of vasodilation is the L-arginine-NO system. Healthy aging has been shown to be associated not only with decreased total body production of NO[37] but also decreased responsiveness to NO.[18,24,38,39] This combination of reduced resistance vessel responsiveness to catecholamines and α_1-adrenergic receptor antagonism results in orthostasis in older people.[40,41] This explains the presence of combined isolated systolic hypertension and orthostatic hypotension in older patients.

Oxidative Stress

The production of ROS causes impairment of the normal endothelial functions. ROS has been implicated in degrading NO, impairing the function of EPC, and disrupting the endothelial homeostasis (**Fig. 3**). In younger people, antioxidants and reactive oxygen scavengers help to minimize the impact that ROS has on the biochemical pathways. With age, the increased production of ROS begins to overwhelm some of those protective mechanisms and the side effects lead to oxidative stress of the endothelium.

Production of Reactive Oxygen Species

- eNOS uncoupling, which is caused by ROS, also produces more reactive oxygen, which potentiates a damaging cycle.
- Nicotinamide adenine dinucleotide phosphate (NADPH) oxidase and xanthine oxidase are both ROS producers.[32] NADPH has been discovered in higher concentrations in the microvasculature of older subjects, and inhibiting this enzyme has been shown to improve endothelial function. Xanthine oxidase also has been associated with increased levels of oxidative stress; however, this has been demonstrated only in the laboratory setting.

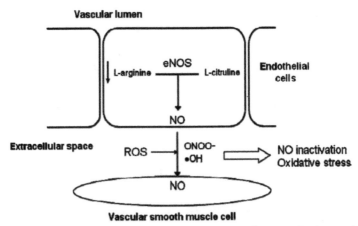

Fig. 3. Cellular signaling pathways that lead to inhibition of NO production and ROS production due to oxidative stress. eNOS catalyzes the production of NO from its precursor L-arginine. ROS located in the extracellular space defunctionalize NO and mitigate its vasodilatory effects on the vascular smooth muscle cell. (*From* Marin C. Endothelial aging associated with oxidative stress can be modulated by a healthy Mediterranean diet. Int J Mol Sci 2013;14(5):8875; with permission.)

- Poorly functioning mitochondria in advanced age produce malfunctioning proteins that increase ROS production.[3]

Reduced Function of Endothelial Progenitor Cells

Since their discovery 20 years ago, there has been growing interest in EPCs and their pivotal role in the maintenance of the endothelial integrity of arteries. These cells are derived from bone marrow and are intimately involved in the repair of injured endothelium and angiogenesis. It has been argued that the decreased availability and function of EPCs that occurs with age leaves the endothelium at higher risk for the development and progression of atherosclerosis.[42] EPCs under normal conditions will migrate to areas of arterial insult and are able to regenerate the endothelial lining. In fact, a surge in EPCs has been demonstrated in patients who are progressing through an acute medical issue, such as a trauma, burn, or surgery. Without an appropriate number of circulating EPCs, these areas of insult will be targets for platelet aggregation and plaque formation. Studies have shown that a lower number of EPCs in otherwise healthy individuals caused a statistically significant decrease in flow-mediated brachial reactivity, which is a marker for endothelial function.[43] Other studies have shown that age does not affect the number of available EPCs in the endothelium, but rather the qualitative function is declined in older individuals.[44] Either way, there are many factors that cause inadequate EPC maintenance of the endothelium, which ultimately result in vascular disease (**Fig. 4**).

Causes of Endothelial Progenitor Cell Depletion and Dysfunction

- ROS cause direct cellular damage to EPCs. EPCs taken from older individuals were found to have a lower amount of antioxidants available, thereby making them more susceptible to reactive oxygen injury.[33]
- As previously discussed, the bioavailability of NO also decreases with age and EPCs are dependent on NO for cell signaling and maintenance.
- Estrogens have been linked to EPC proliferation and postmenopausal women have been shown to have lower levels of these progenitor cells.[45]
- Chronic inflammation is mediated by proinflammatory agents, namely tumor necrosis factor (TNF)-alpha, which has been shown to cause early death to EPCs.[42]
- Higher levels of low-density lipoprotein (LDL) have been implicated in lowering the number of circulating EPCs.[42]
- One study hypothesizes that there is a finite number of EPCs, and once this pool of cells is depleted, the endothelium repair mechanism will be compromised. Patients who had other risk factors for cardiovascular disease had depleted levels of EPCs, which was attributed to EPC exhaustion from increased frequency of endothelial injury.[44]

POTENTIAL TREATMENTS

As the number of people around the world living into their ninth and tenth decades continues to increase, so too will the incidences of cardiovascular-related health problems. It has become clear through previous investigations that patients at higher risk are those with comorbidities that include hypertension, diabetes, hyperlipidemia, renal failure, and smoking. However, there is a subset of elderly patients who are free of these established cardiovascular risk factors, and yet still develop many of the similar problems of progressive atherosclerosis and poor tissue perfusion. As a result, many recent studies have focused on targeting the biochemical pathways that are affected

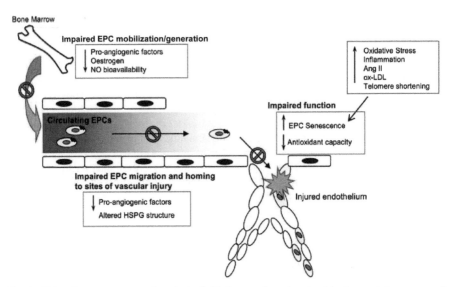

Fig. 4. EPCs migrate to areas of endothelial injury and are involved in the maintenance and repair of the endothelium. Many factors are involved that counter the effect of EPCs. NO induces the generation of EPCs from the bone marrow. Low levels of heparan sulfate proteoglycan (HSPG) or proangiogenic factors impair the EPCs from migrating to the site of injured endothelium. Angiotensin II (Ang II) and LDL increase inflammation and oxidative stress. (*From* Williamson K, Stringer SE. Endothelial progenitor cells enter the aging arena. Front Physiol 2012;3(30):4; with permission.)

by the natural process of aging in an attempt to prolong the health of the vascular system.

Increasing bioavailability of NO has shown some promising results in both experimental and clinical settings. Several drug classes have been shown to alter large-vessel compliance. These include calcium channel blockers, angiotensin-converting enzyme inhibitors, (oral) nitrates, statins, and the potassium channel–opening agent Nicorandil.

Exercise

Not surprisingly, exercise has been associated with a decrease in cardiovascular morbidity and mortality in the elderly. Aside from the more obvious benefits of daily exercise, such as better control of hyperlipidemia, diabetes, and weight loss, exercise also causes alterations at a molecular level that help to improve endothelial function.[43]

- Exercise increases bioavailability of NO and a reduction in the presence of ROS.
- It reduces inflammatory agents such as TNF-alpha.
- Mitochondrial function is improved with exercise, which can promote formation of antioxidants while decreasing the release of ROS as a by-product.
- Studies also suggest that exercise enhances the performance and concentration of EPCs.

Caloric Restriction

Caloric restriction has been shown to promote improved health of the endothelium. The more obvious benefits are a result from a decreased intake of lipid-rich foods, but there are other pathways that have been discovered in previous studies.[29,32]

- Caloric restriction improves the function of the endothelium by stimulating the production of eNOS, thereby increasing the bioavailability of NO.
- It decreases the activity of ROS, which helps to prevent oxidative stress to the endothelium.
- Anti-inflammatory properties are demonstrated with caloric restriction, such as a reduction in TNF-alpha, which helps to mitigate the process of atherosclerosis.

Diet

Studies have looked at the effects of a Mediterranean diet rich in fish and white meat, olive oil, and fruits and vegetables on the vascular system.[33] The results indicate an increase in the bioavailability of NO and improved function and number of EPCs at the level of the endothelium. These foods are high in antioxidants, which can account for the decreased negative effects of ROS.

Supplementation of inorganic nitrite in diets has been shown to induce vascular relaxation and lower blood pressure. A traditional Japanese diet for 10 days increased plasma levels of nitrite and decreased blood pressure in healthy volunteers.[46–49] The longevity enjoyed by the Japanese may be related to high levels of nitrites in their diet. However, concerns regarding the safety of nitrites has precluded widespread clinical interventions.

Statins

Statins increase NO bioavailability by increasing eNOS expression and posttranscriptional modifications, eNOS recoupling, and reduced NO breakdown by ROS.[3] Atorvastatin has been shown to upregulate endothelial cell expression of nNOS in the in vitro setting. In animal models, statins reversed impaired endothelium-dependent vasodilation in old rats and increased eNOS levels. Furthermore, statins increase BH_4 bioavailability and upregulate guanosine triphosphate cyclohydrolase-1, resulting in eNOS recoupling and NO generation in endothelium. In humans, improvement of flow-mediated dilation in the brachial artery and restored BH_4 levels in mammary arteries was noted.[50]

These findings may explain successful outcomes reported with the use of statins in patients with atherosclerotic diseases.[51–53]

Estrogen Replacement

Estrogen has long been linked to improved cardiovascular health, due to the relationship of increased prevalence of atherosclerosis in women after menopause. Estrogen is thought to have endothelial protective properties during the fertile years of the healthy woman.[54]

- Estrogens stimulate enzymes, such as superoxide dismutase, which act to counter the effects of ROS and reduce free radical injury to the endothelium, while also enhancing NOS productivity, which increases the concentration of NO (**Fig. 5**).
- Estrogens have anti-inflammatory properties and have been shown to inhibit the function of COX and thromboxane.
- Matrix metalloproteinases are stimulated by estrogens, which improve the compliance of arteries by decreasing the density of collagen in the wall.

Testosterone Replacement

The decline in vascular function with age has been attributed to the progressive decline in testosterone levels in men over time. Studies have looked at the role of testosterone in the key signaling pathways of endothelial maintenance. These studies have investigated any potential benefits for testosterone replacement in the older male population.

- Testosterone replacement has been shown to improve hyperlipidemia, and studies have described improvements in pulse wave velocities with higher testosterone levels.[55]
- It may increase the bioavailability of NO and improve the function of EPCs.
- Testosterone replacement, however, has been shown to worsen hypertension and lead to renal dysfunction, and its clinical applications for vascular health remain controversial.

INSULINLIKE GROWTH FACTOR

Insulinlike growth factor (IGF) has been demonstrated to enhance the function of the cellular maintenance of the endothelium. Given as a supplement, it can have similar positive effects as seen in other hormone replacement therapy, such as estrogen or testosterone. IGF replacement, however, also has been shown to increase the risk of breast, prostate, and colon cancer, and its role in the prevention of vascular aging needs further investigation.

- Studies have shown that subjects who were treated with IGF had improved function and proliferation of EPCs compared with the control group.[56] This was demonstrated with improved angiogenesis and mobilization of the EPCs to the endothelium.

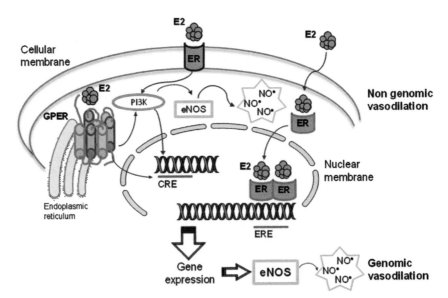

Fig. 5. Schematic of the pathways by which estrogen (E2) increases the bioavailability of NO. Estrogen receptors (ER) bind estrogen and are then stimulated by estrogen-response element (ERE) to increase the gene expression for eNOS production. E2 also interacts with G protein-coupled estrogen receptor (GPER), which increases the expression of cAMP-response element (CRE), thereby augmenting eNOS production by an alteration in DNA signaling. (*From* Novella S, Dantas AP, Segarra G, et al. Vascular aging in women: is estrogen the fountain of youth? Front Physiol 2012;3(165):3; with permission.)

- It has been shown to increase the actions of eNOS, which enhances the bioavailability of NO.
- Other studies have demonstrated IGF to be involved in reducing ROS formation and stimulating antioxidant production (**Fig. 6**).

Oral L-Arginine

Studies have investigated the effects of supplementing L-arginine to increase the substrate for increased NO availability and ultimately improve endothelial function. One study looked at healthy, nonsmoking subjects older than 70 years and found that they had an increased level of ADMA, which leads to inhibition of NOS.[35] After supplementing with L-arginine, a more normal ratio of NOS was available for the production of NO. These subjects had flow-mediated dilation studies performed of the brachial artery before and after supplementation, and were found to have a statistically significant increase in vessel diameter. The conclusion was that increasing the substrate for NO can improve endothelial function of the aging vascular system.

FUTURE DIRECTIONS

There are several new drugs being investigated in research trials that aim to enhance the function of the endothelium by targeting specific biochemical pathways that have been shown to be factors in the process of vascular aging.

Resveratrol

- Resveratrol is a polyphenol synthetic drug that is designed to improve endothelial function by the same mechanism as is seen with caloric restriction.[57,58] Resveratrol also is found in high concentrations in the Mediterranean-style diets, which have been shown to be vasoprotective.
- Resveratrol improves mitochondrial function, reduces free radical formation, increases NO bioavailability by stimulating eNOS, and acts as an anti-inflammatory.

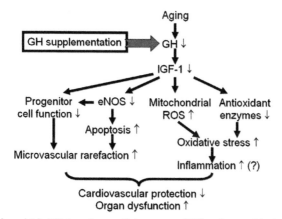

Fig. 6. Pathway by which IGF-1 and growth hormone (GH) reduce oxidative stress and ROS, while promoting the function and availability of eNOS. (*From* Ungvari Z. Mechanisms of vascular aging: new perspectives. J Gerontol A Biol Sci Med Sci 2010;65(10):1036; with permission.)

Sirtuins

- Sirtuins are a class of drug that also target the signaling pathway that is modified by a calorie-restricted diet. Sirtuins are designed to upregulate the expression of Sirt1, which has been shown to improve endothelial viability and longevity, and reduce injury from oxidative species.[32]
- Sirtuins also reduce smooth muscle cell proliferation and can prevent intimal hyperplasia and vessel narrowing.

Rapamycin and Mammalian Target of Rapamycin Complex 1–S6 Kinase 1 Signaling

- Mammalian target of rapamycin complex 1 (mTORC1) is a protein kinase that is involved in the regulation of cellular growth and metabolism.[57] It is thought to play a role in insulin resistance and is seen in higher concentration of older arterial walls.
- Rapamycin inhibits the mTORC1–S6 Kinase 1 (S6K1) signaling pathway, which has been shown to enhance NO bioavailability and decrease ROS.
- Rapamycin also inhibits cell adhesion molecules from lining the arterial walls, which aids in the prevention of thrombosis.
- Resveratrol also has been shown to have inhibitory effects on mTORC1-S6K1 signaling.

SUMMARY

Cardiovascular diseases have become a major cause of morbidity and mortality and are likely to only increase as the elderly population continues to grow. Much is already known about the basic risk factors associated with vascular aging, but there is a new direction of investigation into the health and viability of the endothelium at a biochemical level. Clearly, pathways such as the function of EPCs and concentration of NO play pivotal roles in the maintenance of a healthy endothelium. Discovering a decline in these functions with age opens the door to an entirely new arena of possible treatment interventions designed to counter the effects of natural aging on the vascular system. Most of these investigations are in their infancy and have been demonstrated only in the laboratory setting, but the potential for improving the cardiovascular health of our aging population is vast. As we continue to shift much of our health care focus into prevention tactics and techniques, slowing or reversing the aging process of the vascular system could have a profound impact on our aging population.

REFERENCES

1. Gragasin FS, Bourque SL, Davidge ST. Vascular aging and hemodynamic stability in the intraoperative period. Front Physiol 2012;3:31–7.
2. Ferrari AU, Radaelli A, Centola M. Invited review: aging and the cardiovascular system. J Appl Physiol (1985) 2003;95(6):2591–7.
3. Cau S, Carneiro FS. Differential modulation of nitric oxide synthases in aging: therapeutic opportunities. Front Physiol 2012;3(218):1–11.
4. Mirea O, Donoiu I, Plesea IE. Arterial aging: a brief review. Rom J Morphol Embryol 2012;53(3):473–7.
5. Lekontseva O, Jiang Y, Schleppe C, et al. Altered neuronal nitric oxide synthase in the aging vascular system: implications for estrogens therapy. Endocrinology 2012;153(8):3940–8.
6. Fujiyama S, Amano K, Uehira K, et al. Bone marrow monocyte lineage cells adhere on injured endothelium in a monocyte chemoattractant protein-1-dependent

manner and accelerate reendothelialization as endothelial progenitor cells. Circ Res 2003;93(10):980–9.

7. Keymel S, Kalka C, Rassaf T, et al. Impaired endothelial progenitor cell function predicts age-dependent carotid intimal thickening. Basic Res Cardiol 2008; 103(6):582–6.

8. Virmani R, Avolio AP, Mergner WJ, et al. Effect of aging on aortic morphology in populations with high and low prevalence of hypertension and atherosclerosis. Comparison between occidental and Chinese communities. Am J Pathol 1991; 139(5):1119–29.

9. Benetos A, Waeber B, Izzo J, et al. Influence of age, risk factors, and cardiovascular and renal disease on arterial stiffness: clinical applications. Am J Hypertens 2002;15(12):1101–8.

10. Choi SY, Oh BH, Bae PJ, et al. Age-associated increase in arterial stiffness measured according to the cardio-ankle vascular index without blood pressure changes in healthy adults. J Atheroscler Thromb 2013;20(12):911–23.

11. Li Z, Froehlich J, Galis ZS, et al. Increased expression of matrix metalloproteinase-2 in the thickened intima of aged rats. Hypertension 1999;33(1):116–23.

12. Franklin SS, Gustin W, Wong ND, et al. Hemodynamic patterns of age-related changes in blood pressure. The Framingham Heart Study. Circulation 1997; 96(1):308–15.

13. Blacher J, Asmar R, Djane S, et al. Aortic pulse wave velocity as a marker of cardiovascular risk in hypertensive patients. Hypertension 1999;33(5):1111–7.

14. Blacher J, London GM, Safar ME, et al. Influence of age and end-stage renal disease on the stiffness of carotid wall material in hypertension. J Hypertens 1999;17(2):237–44.

15. Vallance P. Control of the human cardiovascular system by nitric oxide. J Hum Hypertens 1996;10(6):377–81.

16. Wilkinson IB, Qasem A, McEniery CM, et al. Nitric oxide regulates local arterial distensibility in vivo. Circulation 2002;105(2):213–7.

17. Furchgott RF, Zawadzki JV. The obligatory role of endothelial cells in the relaxation of arterial smooth muscle by acetylcholine. Nature 1980;288(27):373–6.

18. Moncada S, Radomski MW, Palmer RM. Endothelium-derived relaxing factor. Identification as nitric oxide and role in the control of vascular tone and platelet function. Biochem Pharmacol 1988;37(13):2495–501.

19. Melikian N, Seddon MD, Casadei B, et al. Neuronal nitric oxide synthase and human vascular regulation. Trends Cardiovasc Med 2009;19(8):256–62.

20. Villanueva C, Giulivi C. Subcellular and cellular locations of nitric oxide synthase isoforms as determinants of health and disease. Free Radic Biol Med 2010;49(3): 307–16.

21. Hecker M, Cattaruzza M, Wagner AH. Regulation of inducible nitric oxide synthase gene expression in vascular smooth muscle cells. Gen Pharmacol 1999;32(1):9–16.

22. Blackwell KA, Sorenson JP, Richardson DM, et al. Mechanisms of aging-induced impairment of endothelium-dependent relaxation: role of tetrahydrobiopterin. Am J Physiol Heart Circ Physiol 2004;287(6):H2448–53.

23. Delp MD, Behnke BJ, Spier SA, et al. Ageing diminishes endothelium-dependent vasodilatation and tetrahydrobiopterin content in rat skeletal muscle arterioles. J Physiol 2008;586(4):1161–8.

24. Gerhard M, Roddy MA, Creager SJ, et al. Aging progressively impairs endothelium-dependent vasodilation in forearm resistance vessels of humans. Hypertension 1996;27(4):849–53.

25. Muller-Delp JM, Spier SA, Ramsey MW, et al. Aging impairs endothelium-dependent vasodilation in rat skeletal muscle arterioles. Am J Physiol Heart Circ Physiol 2002;283(4):H1662–72.

26. Rodriguez-Manas L, El-Assar M, Vallejo S, et al. Endothelial dysfunction in aged humans is related with oxidative stress and vascular inflammation. Aging Cell 2009;8(3):226–38.

27. Sun D, Huang A, Yan EH, et al. Reduced release of nitric oxide to shear stress in mesenteric arteries of aged rats. Am J Physiol Heart Circ Physiol 2004;286(6):H2249–56.

28. Taddei S, Virdis A, Ghiadoni L, et al. Age-related reduction of NO availability and oxidative stress in humans. Hypertension 2001;38(2):274–9.

29. Ungvari Z, Csiszar A, Kaley G. Vascular inflammation in aging. Herz 2004;29(8):733–40.

30. Briones AM, Montoya N, Giraldo J, et al. Ageing affects nitric oxide synthase, cyclooxygenase and oxidative stress enzymes expression differently in mesenteric resistance arteries. Auton Autacoid Pharmacol 2005;25(4):155–62.

31. Novensa L, Novella S, Medina P, et al. Aging negatively affects estrogens-mediated effects on nitric oxide bioavailability by shifting ERalpha/ERbeta balance in female mice. PLoS One 2011;6(9):e25335.

32. El Assar M, Angulo J, Vallejo S, et al. Mechanisms involved in the aging-induced vascular dysfunction. Front Physiol 2012;3(132):1–13.

33. Marin C, Yubero-Serrano EM, Lopez-Miranda J, et al. Endothelial aging associated with oxidative stress can be modulated by a healthy Mediterranean diet. Int J Mol Sci 2013;14(5):8869–89.

34. Marin J, Rodriguez-Martinez MA. Nitric oxide, oxygen-derived free radicals and vascular endothelium [review]. J Auton Pharmacol 1995;15(4):279–307.

35. Bode-Boger SM, Muke J, Surdacki A, et al. Oral L-arginine improves endothelial function in healthy individuals older than 70 years. Vasc Med 2003;8(2):77–81.

36. Elliott HL, Sumner DJ, McLean K, et al. Effect of age on the responsiveness of vascular alpha-adrenoceptors in man. J Cardiovasc Pharmacol 1982;4(3):388–92.

37. Lyons D, Roy S, Patel M, et al. Impaired nitric oxide-mediated vasodilatation and total body nitric oxide production in healthy old age. Clin Sci (Lond) 1997;93(6):519–25.

38. Egashira K, Inou T, Hirooka Y, et al. Effects of age on endothelium-dependent vasodilation of resistance coronary artery by acetylcholine in humans. Circulation 1993;88(1):77–81.

39. Palmer RM, Ashton DS, Moncada S. Vascular endothelial cells synthesize nitric oxide from L-arginine. Nature 1988;333(6174):664–6.

40. Andros E, Detmar-Hanna D, Suteparuk S, et al. The effect of aging on the pharmacokinetics and pharmacodynamics of prazosin. Eur J Clin Pharmacol 1996;50(1–2):41–6.

41. Tsujii T. Comparison of prazosin, terazosin and tamsulosin in the treatment of symptomatic benign prostatic hyperplasia: a short-term open, randomized multicenter study. BPH Medical Therapy Study Group. Benign prostatic hyperplasia. Int J Urol 2000;7(6):199–205.

42. Danta AP, Jimenez-Altayo F, Villa E. Vascular aging: facts and factors. Front Physiol 2012;3(325):1–2.

43. Seals DR, Jablonski KL, Donato AJ. Aging and vascular endothelial function in humans. Clin Sci (Lond) 2011;120(9):357–75.

44. Hill JM, Zalos G, Halcox JP, et al. Circulating endothelial progenitor cells, vascular function, and cardiovascular risk. N Engl J Med 2003;348(7):593–600.

45. Williamson K, Stringer SE. Endothelial progenitor cells enter the aging arena. Front Physiol 2012;3(30):1–7.
46. Cosby K, Partovi KS, Crawford JH, et al. Nitrite reduction to nitric oxide by deoxyhemoglobin vasodilates the human circulation. Nat Med 2003;9(12): 1498–505.
47. Kapil V, Milsom AB, Okorie M, et al. Inorganic nitrate supplementation lowers blood pressure in humans: role for nitrite-derived NO. Hypertension 2010;56(2): 274–81.
48. Larsen FJ, Ekblom B, Sahlin K, et al. Effects of dietary nitrate on blood pressure in healthy volunteers. N Engl J Med 2006;355(26):2792–3.
49. Webb AJ, Patel N, Loukogeorgakis S, et al. Acute blood pressure lowering, vasoprotective, and antiplatelet properties of dietary nitrate via bioconversion to nitrite. Hypertension 2008;51(3):784–90.
50. Antoniades C, Bakogiannis C, Leeson P, et al. Rapid, direct effects of statin treatment on arterial redox state and nitric oxide bioavailability in human athero-sclerosis via tetrahydrobiopterin-mediated endothelial nitric oxide synthase coupling. Circulation 2011;124(3):335–45.
51. Foody JM, Rathore SS, Galusha D, et al. Hydroxymethylglutaryl-CoA reductase inhibitors in older persons with acute myocardial infarction: evidence for an age-statin interaction. J Am Geriatr Soc 2006;54(3):421–30.
52. Gransbo K, Melander O, Wallentin L, et al. Cardiovascular and cancer mortality in very elderly post-myocardial infarction patients receiving statin treatment. J Am Coll Cardiol 2010;55(13):1362–9.
53. Shepherd J, Blauw GJ, Murphy MB, et al. Pravastatin in elderly individuals at risk of vascular disease (PROSPER): a randomised controlled trial. Lancet 2002; 360(9346):1623–30.
54. Novella S, Dantas AP, Segarra G, et al. Vascular aging in women: is estrogen the fountain of youth? Front Physiol 2012;3(165):1–8.
55. Lopes RA, Neves KB, Carneiro FS, et al. Testosterone and vascular function in aging. Front Physiol 2012;3(89):1–9.
56. Thum T, Hoeber S, Froese S, et al. Age-dependent impairment of endothelial progenitor cells is corrected by growth-hormone-mediated increase of insulin-like growth-factor-1. Circ Res 2007;100(3):434–43.
57. Ming XF, Montani JP, Yang Z. Perspectives of targeting mTORC1-S6K1 in cardio-vascular aging. Front Physiol 2012;3(5):1–11.
58. Ungvari Z, Kaley G, de Cabo R, et al. Mechanisms of vascular aging: new perspectives. J Gerontol A Biol Sci Med Sci 2010;65(10):1028–41.

The Effect of Aging on Pulmonary Function

Implications for Monitoring and Support of the Surgical and Trauma Patient

Elie Ramly, MD, Haytham M.A. Kaafarani, MD, MPH*, George C. Velmahos, MD, PhD

KEYWORDS

- Aging • Pulmonary function • Perioperative care
- Postoperative pulmonary complications

KEY POINTS

- Age-related anatomic, physiologic, and immunologic changes to the pulmonary system as well as a high prevalence of chronic pulmonary diseases puts the elderly patient at an especially high risk for postoperative pulmonary complications.
- Successful perioperative respiratory care of the elderly patient relies on careful risk assessment and optimization of pulmonary function and support.
- The success of such efforts aimed at preventing and/or mitigating pulmonary complications in the elderly patient depends on a thorough, individualized, yet standardized and evidence-based approach to the care of every patient.

INTRODUCTION

According to the 2010 Census data, 40.3 million, or 13%, of Americans are now aged 65 years or older, forming one of the most rapidly growing proportions[1] of the US population. Not unexpectedly, the geriatric population accounts for a disproportionately large faction of all surgical procedures performed in the United States.[2] This population is particularly vulnerable to pulmonary disease; in fact, lower respiratory tract disease is the third leading cause of death and a significant source of disability[3] in people older than 65. With age, the respiratory system undergoes a combination of anatomic, physiologic, and immunologic changes[4,5] modulated by cumulative exposure to environmental stress, airborne toxins, cigarette smoke, and infectious agents.[4]

Division of Trauma, Emergency Surgery, and Surgical Critical Care, Massachusetts General Hospital, Harvard Medical School, 165 Cambridge Street, Suite 810, Boston, MA 02114, USA
* Corresponding author.
E-mail address: hkaafarani@mgh.harvard.edu

Surg Clin N Am 95 (2015) 53–69
http://dx.doi.org/10.1016/j.suc.2014.09.009   surgical.theclinics.com
0039-6109/15/$ – see front matter © 2015 Elsevier Inc. All rights reserved.

A better understanding of these interrelated changes not only provides insight into the mechanisms of respiratory impairment and disease in the geriatric population, but also helps clinicians better prepare for, prevent, or mitigate the effects of perioperative or posttrauma pulmonary complications.

THE ANATOMIC AGE-RELATED RESPIRATORY CHANGES

Age affects the pulmonary system by inducing changes in the chest wall, lung parenchyma, and the airway. **Table 1** summarizes the pulmonary anatomic changes observed with age.

Chest Wall

With age, the chest wall undergoes characteristic structural changes that directly affect respiratory function, such as narrowing of the thoracic intervertebral disk spaces. Known as kyphosis,[6] the increase in curvature of the spine results in narrowing of the intercostal space, which in turn decreases the length and alters the angle of insertion of the intercostal muscle fibers, contributing to decreased efficiency and mobility of an already smaller chest cavity.[7] The increase in vertebral angle is clinically associated with a significant decline in the fraction of exhaled volume in 1 second (FEV1) and vital capacity (VC), as described by Lombardi and colleagues.[8] In addition to the mechanical and structural constraints imposed by the aging bony scaffold, intrinsic skeletal muscle mass and strength diminish considerably with age, a process known as sarcopenia.[9] Loss of type II fast-twitch muscle fibers[10] results in attenuated electromyographic activity[11] and a weaker diaphragmatic inspiratory effort, and the decrease in mitochondrial ATP reserve impedes the lung's ability to meet any sudden increases in metabolic demand.[12] Therefore, not only do elderly patients with respiratory disease or those subjected to physiologic stress have an increased metabolic demand in the setting of unfavorable functional anatomy and increased work of breathing, but they also have less ability to respond to the increased stress. This puts the geriatric population at a significantly higher risk for respiratory fatigue and failure,[5,13] and contributes to the difficulty in weaning an elderly patient from the ventilator in the intensive care unit.[14]

Parenchyma

The increased stiffness of the chest wall occurs in parallel with an increase in lung compliance due to loss of lung parenchymal elasticity.[14,15] With aging, there is alteration in the spatial arrangement and cross-linking of parenchymal elastic fibers, which results in gradual reduction in lung elastic recoil, homogeneous enlargement of air spaces, and reduction in alveolar surface area.[14] This functional "senile emphysema" is accompanied by an age-related change in surfactant composition.[16] The ability to

| Table 1 |||
| Anatomic pulmonary age-related changes |||
Chest Wall	**Lung Parenchyma**	**Airway**
↓ Intervertebral disk spaces	↓ Internal elastic recoil	↑ Rigidity of the cervical joints
↑ Kyphosis of the spine	↑ Compliance	↓ Thyromental distance
↓ Intercostal muscle strength	↑ Emphysematous changes	↓ Interincisor gap
↓ Diaphragmatic strength	↑ Mucociliary dysfunction	↑ Mallampati score

↑, increase; ↓, decrease.

clear mucus and particles from the lungs is decreased due to the combined effects of the sarcopenia-induced reduction in cough strength and the aging-induced dysfunction of the mucociliary escalator of both the upper and lower airway.[17,18]

Airway

Elderly patients tend to have a shorter thyromental distance, a smaller interincisor gap, and a high Mallampati score[19–21]; therefore, endotracheal intubation could be more challenging in this patient population.[19] In addition, they often suffer from poor dentition and cervical joint rigidity due to degenerative changes, and may be more difficult to ventilate with a mask.

THE PHYSIOLOGIC AGE-RELATED PULMONARY CHANGES

The pulmonary physiologic changes that occur with age are best described in terms of their effect on lung volumes, gas exchange, and respiratory effort. **Table 2** summarizes the pulmonary physiologic changes observed with age.

Lung Volumes

In the elderly patient, the more rigid chest wall generates less outward force, whereas the more compliant lung allows less inward elastic recoil, resulting in a relatively unchanged total lung capacity.[4,14] On the contrary, the changes affecting the parenchyma occur at a faster rate, leading to air trapping and hyperinflation, increasing residual volume by 5% to 10% per decade and functional residual capacity (FRC) by 1% to 3% per decade.[22] This results in a decrease in VC. The loss of elasticity causes an increase in the "closing volume" or lung volume above which there is premature collapse of small airways.[4]

Both FEV1 and forced vital capacity (FVC) decline by up to 30 mL per year in both men and women, as observed in longitudinal spirometric studies.[23] Chronic smoking accelerates these age-related changes.[24] This expiratory flow limitation contributes to the process of dynamic hyperinflation during exercise; the higher residual volume blunts the curvature of the aging diaphragm, negatively affecting its length-tension relationship and further reducing its already weakened force-generating capacity.[4,25]

Table 2 Physiologic age-related changes		
Lung Volumes	**Gas Exchange**	**Respiratory Drive**
↑↓ TLC unchanged	↑ V/Q mismatch	↓ Central ventilator control
↑ RV	↑ Pulmonary vascular resistance	↑ Central sleep apnea
↑ FRC	↓ Decreased DLCO	↓ Peripheral chemoreceptor and mechanoreceptor signaling
↓ VC	↓ Decreased Pao$_2$	↓ Decreased response to hypoxemia
↓ FEV1; ↓ FVC	↑ Dead space ventilation, ↑ minute ventilation	↓ Decreased response to hypercapnia

↑, Increase; ↓, Decrease; ↑↓, No significant change.
  Abbreviations: DLCO, diffusing lung capacity for carbon monoxide; FEV1, fraction of exhaled volume in 1 second; FRC, functional residual capacity; FVC, forced vital capacity; Pao$_2$, the arterial tension for oxygen; RV, residual volume; TLC, total lung capacity; VC, vital capacity; V/Q, ratio of ventilation to perfusion.

Gas Exchange

Two parameters normally determine gas exchange: ventilation-perfusion (V/Q) matching/ratio and diffusion capacity across the alveolar–capillary interface. Both of those parameters are substantially affected by aging of the respiratory system.[15,26,27]

Mismatch of ratio of ventilation to perfusion

The increase in the closing volume and premature collapse of the small airways[15] particularly in the better-perfused dependent portions of the lung, combined with the age-related heterogeneous changes in the pulmonary circulation, result in a heterogeneous distribution of V/Q ratios across lung units.[26,28] The effect of the ventilation-perfusion mismatch is more pronounced in the supine versus sitting position.[29]

Pulmonary vascular resistance and pressure

An age-related increase in pulmonary vascular resistance is most likely at the origin of an observed 1 mm per decade incremental increase in pulmonary arterial systolic pressure, resulting in pulmonary pressures as high as 40 mm Hg in individuals older than 50 years.[30] Such increase in pulmonary pressures can have serious sequelae, especially in patients at high risk for right-sided cardiac dysfunction.

Diffusion capacity across the alveolar-capillary surface

A decline in the alveolar surface area and in the density of lung capillaries may explain the 5% per decade decrease in the diffusing lung capacity for carbon monoxide (DLCO).[27,31] Healthy older individuals can have up to 50% reduction in the DLCO relative to younger persons.[27] While the arterial tension for oxygen (Pa_{O_2}) declines with age, O_2 saturation remains relatively normal as a virtue of the nature and shape of the oxygen-hemoglobin dissociation curve. This relationship explains the precipitous drop in Pa_{O_2} for adults subjected to increased oxygen demand (eg, during exercise)[32] and the occurrence of hypoxia at high altitude in older adults otherwise nonhypoxic at sea level.[33]

Dead space ventilation

Because of the anatomic and mechanical pulmonary changes that occur with aging, maintenance of a normal Pa_{CO_2} level becomes dependent on an increase in total minute ventilation, which is the sum of alveolar ventilation (VA) and dead space ventilation (VD). The age-related V/Q mismatch described previously results in an increase in VD, a phenomenon made even worse during exercise by the age-related reduction in cardiac output. At peak exercise, VD is 2.5 times higher in older versus younger individuals.[32] Therefore, the increase in VD forces an increase in total minute ventilation to preserve VA. This means that, despite an apparently normal Pa_{CO_2}, the elderly patient has a reduced ventilator reserve due to a constantly higher ventilatory requirement.

Respiratory Drive

Healthy adults older than 65 have a significantly reduced response to hypoxia and hypercapnia relative to younger subjects, signaling the loss of protective respiratory driving mechanisms.[34] This may be partly explained by age-related changes in central ventilatory control, as suggested by the higher prevalence of central sleep apnea among elderly people. Loss of central control is potentially attributable to a reduction in the number of medullary ventral respiratory neurons.[35] In addition, the ability of peripheral mechanoreceptors and chemoreceptors in the chest wall and lung parenchyma to perceive methacholine-provoked bronchoconstriction and associated reduction in lung function significantly decreases with age.[4,14]

THE IMMUNOLOGIC AGE-RELATED PULMONARY CHANGES

The immunologic changes observed with age happen at the level of proinflammatory immune mediators as well as the innate and adaptive immunity.

Immune Mediators

Aging is associated with systemic immune dysfunction known as "inflamm-aging", often manifesting as increased levels of tissue and circulating proinflammatory cytokines[36–38] (eg, interleukins IL-1β and IL-6, tumor necrosis factor-α) in the absence of an immunologic threat, as well as concomitant "immunosenescence" or a blunted response to pathogenic threat or tissue injury.[5,39] The 2 phenomena are closely related, and the imbalance in immune mediators, which results in a proinflammatory state at baseline seems to play a role in the age-related destruction of lung parenchyma.[5]

Innate and Adaptive Immunity

Toll-like receptors (TLRs) are important elements in the initiation of the innate immune response. With age, murine and human TLR expression is reduced and the resultant downstream signaling is altered in monocytes and macrophages.[40–42] Similar to all macrophages, the cytotoxic activity of alveolar macrophages is also reduced. In addition, the alveolar macrophages of older individuals display fewer reactive oxygen species (ROS) in response to lipopolysaccharide exposure, and their neutrophils produce less superoxide,[5] resulting in a suboptimal response to infectious agents.

Adaptive immunity also is affected by aging. In animal studies, dendritic cells have been found to have poor migration to lymph nodes and decreased subsequent T-cell activation with advanced age.[43] The thymus, where naïve T cells are produced, is replaced by fatty tissue by age 60 in humans.[44] This results in an increase in the ratio of memory T cells to naïve (both CD4+ and CD8+) T cells. This in turn reduces the magnitude of the adaptive immune response that can be mounted against a new infection.[45–47] Similarly, with age, B cells have a reduced antibody-secreting capacity,[48] subsequently resulting in a less-effective antigen-specific response. The reduced effectiveness of both innate and adaptive immune responses accounts for the vulnerability of elderly patients to respiratory pathogens and injury.

PREEXISTING PULMONARY COMORBIDITIES IN THE ELDERLY SURGICAL OR TRAUMA PATIENT

The age-related decline in pulmonary function observed in elderly patients is often accompanied by debilitating cardiac or pulmonary diseases. Many of these diseases are either caused or exacerbated by long-standing cigarette smoking.[49] Of these pulmonary diseases, chronic obstructive pulmonary disease (COPD), emphysema, asthma, obstructive sleep apnea (OSA), and pulmonary edema in the setting of congestive heart failure (CHF) are some of the most commonly encountered in the elderly surgical or trauma patient. Perioperative management of these conditions requires special attention, as they are often associated with an increased risk of postoperative complications.

Chronic Obstructive Pulmonary Disease

The prevalence of COPD in patients aged 65 years and older is at least 10% in the United States.[50] Interpretation of pulmonary function tests (PFTs) needs to take into account the age-related expected decrease in FEV1/FVC ratio. Accordingly, the American Thoracic and European Respiratory Societies recommend using below the 5th percentile of the normal distribution of FEV1/FVC (in addition to clinical assessment) as the cutoff to diagnose COPD in elderly patients rather than the previously used fixed ratio of 0.7.[51,52]

Patients with COPD have an increased risk of postoperative pulmonary complications.[53] Thus, patients' pulmonary function should be optimized before any operation. In addition to continuation of the usual medication regimen, prophylactic treatment with azithromycin has been shown in a recent trial to decrease the frequency of exacerbations, albeit at the expense of slightly increasing the risk of hearing loss and promoting microbial-resistance patterns.[54] Acute COPD exacerbations should be aggressively treated and nonurgent surgery should be deferred, when possible, until the exacerbation has resolved. Inhaled ipratropium, beta-adrenergic–receptor agonists, smoking cessation, and physical therapy, supplemented by antibiotics and inhaled or systemic steroids, can reduce the risk for postoperative pulmonary complications in the patient with COPD.[49] When possible, beta-blockers should be avoided in patients with COPD to avoid potential bronchospasm.[55,56]

Asthma

Asthma prevalence in patients 65 years or older is estimated to be between 4% and 8%; many patients are often misdiagnosed as having COPD. It is important to carefully review a patient's list of medications, as several of the commonly used drugs in elderly people are associated with asthma, particularly beta-blockers, nonsteroidal anti-inflammatory drugs, and postmenopausal hormone replacement therapy.[52] However, in contrast to COPD, the evidence available suggests that asthma is not a strong independent risk factor for postoperative pulmonary complications.[53,57]

Obstructive Sleep Apnea

Age-related weakening of pharyngeal muscular support and upper airway dysfunction contribute to the higher prevalence of OSA observed in elderly patients, especially if they are obese. OSA affects up to 25% of adult general surgical patients, with most being diagnosed during preoperative evaluation. OSA is associated with difficulty in airway management in the immediate perioperative phase, but has not been clearly correlated with pulmonary complications in clinical studies.[53,58] Patients having moderate to severe OSA and comorbidities or undergoing a high-risk surgical procedure may benefit from preoperative and immediate postoperative continuous positive airway pressure (CPAP), although the optimal duration of therapy is yet to be determined.[55,58]

Congestive Heart Failure

CHF and resultant pulmonary edema are major risk factors for perioperative cardiopulmonary complications, especially in the elderly. Nonurgent surgery should be deferred for patients with decompensated or severe CHF (worsening chronic or new-onset CHF; New York Heart Association class IV symptoms). These patients should be instead medically optimized with beta-blockers and angiotensin-converting enzyme inhibitors before any planned surgery. In patients with known controlled CHF, preoperative echocardiographic reassessment of left ventricular function is reasonable, although its benefit is unclear if symptoms have been relatively stable since the last evaluation. The role of brain natriuretic peptide (BNP) and N-terminal proBNP measurements in guiding therapy or predicting perioperative cardiac risk among patients with CHF also remains uncertain.[55,59]

For patients undergoing abdominal surgery, laparoscopy might be less invasive and cause fewer fluid shifts and postoperative ileus postoperatively, but the creation of a pneumoperitoneum intraoperatively can have adverse effects on the hemodynamic and cardiac function of the elderly patient with CHF. Specifically, insufflation of carbon dioxide raises intra-abdominal pressure, thus reducing cardiac output and increasing vascular resistance; both changes can worsen an existing CHF.[60] CHF has been found to significantly increase the risk of postoperative pulmonary complications, such as pulmonary edema, pleural effusion, acute respiratory failure, and the need for mechanical ventilation.[55,56]

PULMONARY COMPLICATIONS IN THE POSTOPERATIVE AND POSTTRAUMA ELDERLY PATIENT

Postoperative pulmonary complications include atelectasis, bronchospasm, aspiration, pneumonia, pulmonary embolism, pleural effusion, and exacerbation of chronic lung disease.[49]

Aspiration and Pneumonia

Diminished respiratory muscle strength and mass, attenuated cough and swallowing reflexes, dysfunction of mucociliary clearance, and derangement of immune mechanisms all put elderly patients at an increased risk for postoperative pulmonary aspiration and pneumonia. This is often exacerbated by coexistent gastroesophageal reflux disease and poor oral hygiene.[5,14] The risk is particularly high in the presence of cerebrovascular or neurologic disease, common conditions in the elderly population. The risk of aspiration is not decreased (and might be worse) with routine use of nasogastric tubes (NGTs) perioperatively; therefore, NGTs should be reserved for selected patients with inability to tolerate oral intake or those having significant abdominal distention and/or vomiting.[61,62]

Pulmonary Embolism

The risk of pulmonary embolism (PE) and its associated mortality increase with age. In addition to the high prevalence of comorbidities and immobility in elderly patients, the role of an independent age-related hypercoagulable state is still unclear.[63] D-dimer levels are commonly elevated in older adults, which is why the conventional screening cutoff value of 500 μg/L should be substituted with an age-adjusted value of "age × 10 μg/L" for higher specificity in patients older than 50.[64,65] Computed tomography and pulmonary angiography, the 2 standard diagnostic modalities, are to be used with special caution in the geriatric population in view of the high prevalence of kidney dysfunction that could be worsened with intravenous contrast administration. Eligible elderly patients should receive pharmacologic and/or mechanical deep vein thrombosis prophylaxis, as appropriate; in the event of a PE, anticoagulation or thrombolytic treatment should be administered with no account of age as an independent contraindication. Vena caval filters can be considered when anticoagulation is contraindicated.[66]

PERIOPERATIVE PULMONARY EVALUATION AND OPTIMIZATION OF THE ELDERLY SURGICAL PATIENT

Care of the elderly surgical or trauma patient presents clinical challenges in the preoperative, intraoperative, and postoperative phases.

Preoperative Care

Risk stratification

Elderly patients have a higher risk of postoperative pulmonary complications.[57] Assessment of the general health status with special attention to known risk factors and co-morbidities, combined with appropriate laboratory testing and imaging where appropriate is recommended to direct the optimization of respiratory function and better planning of anesthesia and surgery. Two pulmonary risk indices[67,68] to predict postoperative pneumonia and respiratory failure (**Table 3**) have been developed by Arozullah and colleagues based on National Surgical Quality Improvement Project (NSQIP) data. Potential risk factors were entered into a logistic regression model, which allowed for the creation of a scoring system where the point values assigned to each risk factor sum up to a risk index assigned to each patient. Risk factors common to both indices included advanced age, type of surgery including abdominal, thoracic, and emergency surgery, low albumin level or recent weight loss, high blood urea nitrogen level, dependent functional status, and history of COPD.

Other risk factors that have been associated with postoperative pulmonary complications in the elderly include an American Society of Anesthesiologists (ASA) physical status classification of II or greater[53,57] and smoking. There is enough evidence to suggest a modest increase in risk for postoperative pulmonary complications among current smokers,[51] even in the absence of chronic lung disease.[49] Although the prevalence of obesity is high and is increasing in the elderly, obesity by itself has not been consistently found to be an independent risk factor for pulmonary complications, although it does result in lower Pao_2 during wakefulness and under anesthesia due to the reduced chest wall compliance.

Table 3
Postoperative respiratory failure risk index in men after major noncardiac surgery

Preoperative Predictor	Point Value
Type of surgery	
Abdominal aortic aneurysm	27
Thoracic	21
Neurosurgery, upper abdominal, or peripheral vascular	14
Neck	1
Emergency surgery	11
Albumin (<30 g/L)	9
Blood urea nitrogen (>30 mg/dL)	8
Partially or fully dependent functional status	7
History of chronic obstructive pulmonary disease	6
Age (y)	
≥70	6
60–69	4

Class	Point Total	Predicted Probability (%) of Postoperative Respiratory Failure
1	≤10	0.5
2	11–19	2.2
3	20–27	5.0
4	28–40	11.6
5	>40	30.5

Adapted from Arozullah AM, Daley J, Henderson WG, et al. Multifactorial risk index for predicting postoperative respiratory failure in men after major noncardiac surgery. The National Veterans Administration Surgical Quality Improvement Program. Ann Surg 2000;232(2):242–53; with permission.

Pulmonary function testing

PFT is useful in predicting pulmonary function after lung resection. For extrathoracic surgery, the available data regarding its usefulness are mixed. Although a lower FEV1 seems to be predictive of postoperative pulmonary complications, no prohibitive threshold has been consistently reported.[57] We do not recommend routine preoperative PFT and chest radiography to predict a patient's risk for postoperative pulmonary complications; however, PFT may help in preoperative planning and decision-making in the elderly patient with a significant history of COPD or asthma.[53] Preoperative PFT also may be useful to determine the degree of baseline bronchoconstriction in elderly patients with moderate-severe asthma and their therapeutic response to different bronchodilators.

Risk modification

Smoking Smoking cessation counseling is essential, as the risk for postoperative pulmonary complications has been shown to significantly decline with preoperative smoking cessation.[69] However, the optimal number of weeks of perioperative smoking cessation for elective surgery remains unclear.[69–71] Interestingly, some data suggest that stopping cigarette smoking very shortly (rather than several weeks) before surgery may be more harmful than continuing usual smoking habits. This observation may be attributable to selection bias favoring sicker patients in the cessation group or to unfavorable physiologic effects, such as transient increase in cough or sputum in the first 1 to 2 months after cessation.[57,72]

Nutrition Although hypoalbuminemia and malnutrition increase the risk for postoperative pulmonary complications, short-term nutritional supplementation (total parenteral nutrition or total enteral nutrition) has not been consistently shown to improve postoperative outcomes.[53]

Intraoperative Care

Regional versus general anesthesia

Studies on geriatric patients undergoing hip repair and other procedures[73] suggest that spinal anesthesia, compared with general anesthesia, can decrease perioperative mortality, deep vein thrombosis, delirium, myocardial infarction, pneumonia, fatal PE, and hypoxia.[74] An additional advantage to spinal anesthesia is reduction in the amount of opioid analgesics required postoperatively.[73,75] When feasible, regional anesthesia should be chosen for the geriatric patient population.

Anesthetics, sedatives, and neuromuscular blocking agents

As elderly patients often have decreased oropharyngeal reflexes, the use of rapid-sequence anesthetic induction and intubation is usually preferable,[14] but the evidence available regarding decreased incidence of aspiration with this technique is inconclusive.[76] In view of the decreased reserves of elderly patients, a prolonged preoxygenation of up to 3 minutes with 100% oxygen is essential to avoid hypoxia during induction.[77] The alterations in pharmacokinetics and pharmacodynamics that occur with aging should be taken into consideration while determining the doses of anesthetic drugs. The minimum alveolar concentration of all inhalational agents decreases by approximately 6% per decade after age 40.[78–80] Smaller initial doses of anesthetic agents should be used, while allowing for larger intervals between the doses. Long-acting benzodiazepines, such as lorazepam and diazepam should be avoided in elderly individuals, when possible. Excessive narcotic administration also should be avoided, as it could easily precipitate hypoventilation and respiratory acidosis in the elderly patient. The choice of neuromuscular blockers used is equally important, as the rate of complications is higher with the use of long-acting versus short-acting blockers.[81,82] Adequate reversal of the neuromuscular blockade should be checked before any planned extubation, because neuromuscular blocking agents can have prolonged duration of action in elderly patients with decreased liver or renal metabolism. Residual pancuronium neuromuscular blockade has been associated with up to threefold increase in the risk of postoperative pulmonary complications.[81]

Laparoscopic versus open abdominal surgery

Thoracic and upper abdominal surgeries are associated with higher rates of postoperative pulmonary complications.[83] Open upper abdominal surgery is known to result in postoperative reduction in FRC, FVC, and FEV1 by up to 60%, a restrictive pattern caused by both pain and some form of postoperative diaphragmatic dysfunction. Randomized studies have demonstrated better respiratory function after laparoscopic versus open cholecystectomy.[84,85] When feasible and safe, laparoscopy is generally favored over open technique in elderly patients with pulmonary compromise. The benefits of laparoscopy are to be carefully weighed in against the risk of worsening cardiovascular function in the elderly patients with significant CHF or those at high risk for intraoperative hemodynamic instability.

Postoperative Care

Respiratory support

Elderly patients are more likely to develop respiratory failure requiring mechanical ventilation.[13] When possible, noninvasive positive pressure ventilation should be used to avoid endotracheal intubation and mechanical ventilation. CPAP can decrease respiratory complications in patients who develop hypoxemia after major abdominal surgery,[86,87] by increasing mean airway pressure, recruiting collapsed alveoli, increasing minute ventilation, and maintaining upper airway patency. Biphasic positive airway pressure provides additional airway support during inspiration and allows the respiratory muscles to intermittently rest. If noninvasive techniques are not sufficient, endotracheal intubation may be required.

Because elderly patients have compromised respiratory reserves with decreased lung elasticity, FVC respiratory muscle strength, and chest wall compliance,[14] it may be especially difficult to wean them off the mechanical ventilator once instituted.[88] Age is suggested as an independent predictor of higher mortality rates in patients with acute respiratory distress syndrome.[89] Even though early tracheostomy has not been found to decrease the risk of ventilator-associated pneumonia, it might decrease the number of days on mechanical ventilation and should be sought in the elderly patient with persistent respiratory failure.[90]

Lung expansion techniques

Lung expansion techniques include incentive spirometry, chest physical therapy, deep breathing exercises, cough, postural drainage, percussion and vibration, suctioning and ambulation, intermittent positive-pressure breathing, and CPAP.[53] Evidence is lacking on the benefit of any of these methods when used alone or in combination for prophylactic postoperative respiratory therapy. Although incentive spirometry remains widely used, systematic reviews have failed to demonstrate reduction in pulmonary complications after cardiothoracic or abdominal surgery with its use.[91-94] Early mobilization and upright patient positioning help improve gas exchange and pulmonary mechanics in the elderly.[95] CPAP is helpful in more complex cases of respiratory failure.[87]

Postoperative analgesia

Opioids are approximately twice as potent in elderly patients because of decreased clearance and increased brain sensitivity,[96] resulting in an increased risk for perioperative hypoventilation and apnea. A multimodal approach to analgesia should always be used in the elderly patient to reduce opiate requirements. Standing doses of adjunct nonnarcotic pain medication (eg, acetaminophen) should be used when possible. Patient-controlled analgesia (PCA) should be instituted, when possible, as it has been associated with a reduction in the rate of pulmonary complications.[97] In addition, the incorporation of regional techniques, including PCA epidural[98] for elderly patients has been shown to improve postoperative pain control and decrease hospital stay.[99,100] Postoperative epidural analgesia is superior to parenteral narcotics at reducing the rate of pulmonary complications and the need for prolonged ventilation or reintubation. Because it improves postoperative lung function and blood oxygenation,[101] epidural anesthesia should always be considered in elderly patients undergoing thoracic, abdominal, or major vascular surgery.[49] Similarly, new meta-analyses are suggesting that paravertebral anesthesia can provide the same results as epidural anesthesia in patients undergoing major thoracic surgery, while having a better side-effects profile.[102,103] Despite the obvious benefits of regional analgesia in the elderly, it does not seem to confer a significant protective advantage with regard to the rates of postoperative delirium or cognitive decline.[100]

Postoperative delirium

Impaired sensorium or delirium is common after major surgery in the elderly patient population. Postoperative delirium is associated with an increased risk of postoperative respiratory failure and pneumonia after major noncardiac surgery.[57,67,68] Impaired mobility; a higher ASA class; undertreatment of postoperative pain; and administration of benzodiazepines, tramadol, or meperidine, among many other agents, have been associated with postoperative delirium. The type of anesthesia or analgesia technique used does not seem to alter the risk.[104–106] The evidence on whether the prophylactic use of antipsychotics can reduce the risk of postoperative delirium in elderly patients is still nondefinitive.[100,107]

SUMMARY

Elderly patients are a rapidly growing segment of the surgical population. The age-associated anatomic and physiologic changes and high prevalence of chronic diseases affecting the respiratory system place elderly patients at an especially high risk for developing postoperative pulmonary complications. Perioperative respiratory management of these patients starts with a thorough evaluation of their risk factors that can be modified and continues with optimization of their lung function throughout all phases of surgical care. The success of such efforts aimed at preventing and/or mitigating pulmonary complications in the elderly patient depends on a thorough, individualized, yet standardized and evidence-based approach to the care of every patient.

REFERENCES

1. Werner CA. Census 2010 Brief C2010BR-09: the older population: 2010. Washington, DC: US Department of Commerce; 2010.
2. Neuman MD, Bosk CL. The redefinition of aging in American surgery. Milbank Q 2013;91(2):288–315.
3. Minino AM. Death in the United States, 2011. NCHS Data Brief 2013;(115):1–8.

4. Vaz Fragoso CA, Gill TM. Respiratory impairment and the aging lung: a novel paradigm for assessing pulmonary function. J Gerontol A Biol Sci Med Sci 2012;67(3):264–75.

5. Lowery EM, Brubaker AL, Kuhlmann E, et al. The aging lung. Clin Interv Aging 2013;8:1489–96.

6. Bartynski WS, Heller MT, Grahovac SZ, et al. Severe thoracic kyphosis in the older patient in the absence of vertebral fracture: association of extreme curve with age. AJNR Am J Neuroradiol 2005;26(8):2077–85.

7. Culham EG, Jimenez HA, King CE. Thoracic kyphosis, rib mobility, and lung volumes in normal women and women with osteoporosis. Spine 1994;19(11):1250–5.

8. Lombardi I Jr, Oliveira LM, Mayer AF, et al. Evaluation of pulmonary function and quality of life in women with osteoporosis. Osteoporos Int 2005;16(10):1247–53.

9. Brown M, Hasser EM. Complexity of age-related change in skeletal muscle. J Gerontol A Biol Sci Med Sci 1996;51(2):B117–23.

10. Larsson L. Histochemical characteristics of human skeletal muscle during aging. Acta Physiol Scand 1983;117(3):469–71.

11. Polkey MI, Harris ML, Hughes PD, et al. The contractile properties of the elderly human diaphragm. Am J Respir Crit Care Med 1997;155(5):1560–4.

12. Desler C, Hansen TL, Frederiksen JB, et al. Is there a link between mitochondrial reserve respiratory capacity and aging? J Aging Res 2012;2012:192503.

13. Sevransky JE, Haponik EF. Respiratory failure in elderly patients. Clin Geriatr Med 2003;19(1):205–24.

14. Sprung J, Gajic O, Warner DO. Review article: age related alterations in respiratory function—anesthetic considerations. Can J Anaesth 2006;53(12):1244–57.

15. Janssens JP. Aging of the respiratory system: impact on pulmonary function tests and adaptation to exertion. Clin Chest Med 2005;26(3):469–84, vi–vii.

16. Tagaram HR, Wang G, Umstead TM, et al. Characterization of a human surfactant protein A1 (SP-A1) gene-specific antibody; SP-A1 content variation among individuals of varying age and pulmonary health. Am J Physiol Lung Cell Mol Physiol 2007;292(5):L1052–63.

17. de Oliveira-Maul JP, de Carvalho HB, Miyuki Goto D, et al. Aging, diabetes, and hypertension are associated with decreased nasal mucociliary clearance. Chest 2013;143(4):1091–7.

18. Svartengren M, Falk R, Philipson K. Long-term clearance from small airways decreases with age. Eur Respir J 2005;26(4):609–15.

19. Rose DK, Cohen MM. The airway: problems and predictions in 18,500 patients. Can J Anaesth 1994;41(5 Pt 1):372–83.

20. Langeron O, Masso E, Huraux C, et al. Prediction of difficult mask ventilation. Anesthesiology 2000;92(5):1229–36.

21. Moon HY, Baek CW, Kim JS, et al. The causes of difficult tracheal intubation and preoperative assessments in different age groups. Korean J Anesthesiol 2013;64(4):308–14.

22. Zaugg M, Lucchinetti E. Respiratory function in the elderly. Anesthesiol Clin North America 2000;18(1):47–58, vi.

23. Knudson RJ, Slatin RC, Lebowitz MD, et al. The maximal expiratory flow-volume curve. Normal standards, variability, and effects of age. Am Rev Respir Dis 1976;113(5):587–600.

24. Griffith KA, Sherrill DL, Siegel EM, et al. Predictors of loss of lung function in the elderly: the Cardiovascular Health Study. Am J Respir Crit Care Med 2001;163(1):61–8.

25. Polkey MI, Hamnegard CH, Hughes PD, et al. Influence of acute lung volume change on contractile properties of human diaphragm. J Appl Physiol (1985) 1998;85(4):1322–8.

26. Cardus J, Burgos F, Diaz O, et al. Increase in pulmonary ventilation-perfusion inequality with age in healthy individuals. Am J Respir Crit Care Med 1997; 156(2 Pt 1):648–53.

27. Guenard H, Marthan R. Pulmonary gas exchange in elderly subjects. Eur Respir J 1996;9(12):2573–7.

28. Ohlsson J, Middaugh M, Hlastala MP. Reduction of lung perfusion increases VA/Q heterogeneity. J Appl Physiol (1985) 1989;66(5):2423–30.

29. Hardie JA, Morkve O, Ellingsen I. Effect of body position on arterial oxygen tension in the elderly. Respiration 2002;69(2):123–8.

30. McQuillan BM, Picard MH, Leavitt M, et al. Clinical correlates and reference intervals for pulmonary artery systolic pressure among echocardiographically normal subjects. Circulation 2001;104(23):2797–802.

31. Stam H, Hrachovina V, Stijnen T, et al. Diffusing capacity dependent on lung volume and age in normal subjects. J Appl Physiol (1985) 1994;76(6):2356–63.

32. American Thoracic Society, American College of Chest Physicians. ATS/ACCP Statement on cardiopulmonary exercise testing. Am J Respir Crit Care Med 2003;167(2):211–77.

33. Crapo RO, Jensen RL, Hegewald M, et al. Arterial blood gas reference values for sea level and an altitude of 1,400 meters. Am J Respir Crit Care Med 1999;160(5 Pt 1):1525–31.

34. Kronenberg RS, Drage CW. Attenuation of the ventilatory and heart rate responses to hypoxia and hypercapnia with aging in normal men. J Clin Invest 1973;52(8):1812–9.

35. Celle S, Peyron R, Faillenot I, et al. Undiagnosed sleep-related breathing disorders are associated with focal brainstem atrophy in the elderly. Hum Brain Mapp 2009;30(7):2090–7.

36. Kovacs EJ, Grabowski KA, Duffner LA, et al. Survival and cell mediated immunity after burn injury in aged mice. J Am Aging Assoc 2002;25(1):3–9.

37. Gomez CR, Acuna-Castillo C, Nishimura S, et al. Serum from aged F344 rats conditions the activation of young macrophages. Mech Ageing Dev 2006; 127(3):257–63.

38. Ershler WB, Keller ET. Age-associated increased interleukin-6 gene expression, late-life diseases, and frailty. Annu Rev Med 2000;51:245–70.

39. Panda A, Arjona A, Sapey E, et al. Human innate immunosenescence: causes and consequences for immunity in old age. Trends Immunol 2009;30(7): 325–33.

40. Boehmer ED, Meehan MJ, Cutro BT, et al. Aging negatively skews macrophage TLR2- and TLR4-mediated pro-inflammatory responses without affecting the IL-2-stimulated pathway. Mech Ageing Dev 2005;126(12):1305–13.

41. van Duin D, Mohanty S, Thomas V, et al. Age-associated defect in human TLR-1/2 function. J Immunol 2007;178(2):970–5.

42. Renshaw M, Rockwell J, Engleman C, et al. Cutting edge: impaired Toll-like receptor expression and function in aging. J Immunol 2002;169(9):4697–701.

43. Grolleau-Julius A, Harning EK, Abernathy LM, et al. Impaired dendritic cell function in aging leads to defective antitumor immunity. Cancer Res 2008;68(15): 6341–9.

44. Gruver AL, Hudson LL, Sempowski GD. Immunosenescence of ageing. J Pathol 2007;211(2):144–56.

45. Timm JA, Thoman ML. Maturation of CD4+ lymphocytes in the aged microenvironment results in a memory-enriched population. J Immunol 1999;162(2):711–7.
46. Posnett DN, Sinha R, Kabak S, et al. Clonal populations of T cells in normal elderly humans: the T cell equivalent to "benign monoclonal gammapathy". J Exp Med 1994;179(2):609–18.
47. Provinciali M, Moresi R, Donnini A, et al. Reference values for CD4+ and CD8+ T lymphocytes with naive or memory phenotype and their association with mortality in the elderly. Gerontology 2009;55(3):314–21.
48. Song H, Price PW, Cerny J. Age-related changes in antibody repertoire: contribution from T cells. Immunol Rev 1997;160:55–62.
49. Smetana GW. Preoperative pulmonary evaluation. N Engl J Med 1999;340(12): 937–44.
50. Mannino DM, Homa DM, Akinbami LJ, et al. Chronic obstructive pulmonary disease surveillance—United States, 1971-2000. MMWR Surveill Summ 2002; 51(6):1–16.
51. Pellegrino R, Viegi G, Brusasco V, et al. Interpretative strategies for lung function tests. Eur Respir J 2005;26(5):948–68.
52. Akgun KM, Crothers K, Pisani M. Epidemiology and management of common pulmonary diseases in older persons. J Gerontol A Biol Sci Med Sci 2012; 67(3):276–91.
53. Qaseem A, Snow V, Fitterman N, et al, Clinical Efficacy Assessment Subcommittee of the American College of Physicians. Risk assessment for and strategies to reduce perioperative pulmonary complications for patients undergoing noncardiothoracic surgery: a guideline from the American College of Physicians. Ann Intern Med 2006;144:575–80.
54. Albert RK, Connett J, Bailey WC, et al. Azithromycin for prevention of exacerbations of COPD. N Engl J Med 2011;365(8):689–98.
55. Scott IA, Shohag HA, Kam PC, et al. Preoperative cardiac evaluation and management of patients undergoing elective non-cardiac surgery. Med J Aust 2013;199(10):667–73.
56. Mascarenhas J, Azevedo A, Bettencourt P. Coexisting chronic obstructive pulmonary disease and heart failure: implications for treatment, course and mortality. Curr Opin Pulm Med 2010;16(2):106–11.
57. Smetana GW, Lawrence VA, Cornell JE, American College of Physicians. Preoperative pulmonary risk stratification for noncardiothoracic surgery: systematic review for the American College of Physicians. Ann Intern Med 2006;144(8): 581–95.
58. Adesanya AO, Lee W, Greilich NB, et al. Perioperative management of obstructive sleep apnea. Chest 2010;138(6):1489–98.
59. Priebe HJ. Preoperative cardiac management of the patient for non-cardiac surgery: an individualized and evidence-based approach. Br J Anaesth 2011; 107(1):83–96.
60. Bettelli G. Preoperative evaluation in geriatric surgery: comorbidity, functional status and pharmacological history. Minerva Anestesiol 2011;77(6):637–46.
61. Cheatham ML, Chapman WC, Key SP, et al. A meta-analysis of selective versus routine nasogastric decompression after elective laparotomy. Ann Surg 1995; 221(5):469–76 [discussion: 476–8].
62. Nelson R, Tse B, Edwards S. Systematic review of prophylactic nasogastric decompression after abdominal operations. Br J Surg 2005;92(6):673–80.
63. Mari D, Mannucci PM, Coppola R, et al. Hypercoagulability in centenarians: the paradox of successful aging. Blood 1995;85(11):3144–9.

64. Schouten HJ, Geersing GJ, Koek HL, et al. Diagnostic accuracy of conventional or age adjusted D-dimer cut-off values in older patients with suspected venous thromboembolism: systematic review and meta-analysis. BMJ 2013;346:f2492.
65. Righini M, Van Es J, Den Exter PL, et al. Age-adjusted D-dimer cutoff levels to rule out pulmonary embolism: the ADJUST-PE study. JAMA 2014;311(11):1117–24.
66. Berman AR. Pulmonary embolism in the elderly. Clin Geriatr Med 2001;17(1):107–30.
67. Arozullah AM, Daley J, Henderson WG, et al. Multifactorial risk index for predicting postoperative respiratory failure in men after major noncardiac surgery. The National Veterans Administration Surgical Quality Improvement Program. Ann Surg 2000;232(2):242–53.
68. Arozullah AM, Khuri SF, Henderson WG, et al, Participants in the National Veterans Affairs Surgical Quality Improvement Program. Development and validation of a multifactorial risk index for predicting postoperative pneumonia after major noncardiac surgery. Ann Intern Med 2001;135(10):847–57.
69. Warner MA, Offord KP, Warner ME, et al. Role of preoperative cessation of smoking and other factors in postoperative pulmonary complications: a blinded prospective study of coronary artery bypass patients. Mayo Clin Proc 1989;64(6):609–16.
70. Moller AM, Villebro N, Pedersen T, et al. Effect of preoperative smoking intervention on postoperative complications: a randomised clinical trial. Lancet 2002;359(9301):114–7.
71. Nakagawa M, Tanaka H, Tsukuma H, et al. Relationship between the duration of the preoperative smoke-free period and the incidence of postoperative pulmonary complications after pulmonary surgery. Chest 2001;120(3):705–10.
72. Yamashita S, Yamaguchi H, Sakaguchi M, et al. Effect of smoking on intraoperative sputum and postoperative pulmonary complication in minor surgical patients. Respir Med 2004;98(8):760–6.
73. Rodgers A, Walker N, Schug S, et al. Reduction of postoperative mortality and morbidity with epidural or spinal anaesthesia: results from overview of randomised trials. BMJ 2000;321(7275):1493.
74. Luger TJ, Kammerlander C, Gosch M, et al. Neuroaxial versus general anaesthesia in geriatric patients for hip fracture surgery: does it matter? Osteoporos Int 2010;21(Suppl 4):S555–72.
75. Luger TJ, Kammerlander C, Luger MF, et al. Mode of anesthesia, mortality and outcome in geriatric patients. Z Gerontol Geriatr 2014;47(2):110–24.
76. Neilipovitz DT, Crosby ET. No evidence for decreased incidence of aspiration after rapid sequence induction. Can J Anaesth 2007;54(9):748–64.
77. Valentine SJ, Marjot R, Monk CR. Preoxygenation in the elderly: a comparison of the four-maximal-breath and three-minute techniques. Anesth Analg 1990;71(5):516–9.
78. Mapleson WW. Effect of age on MAC in humans: a meta-analysis. Br J Anaesth 1996;76(2):179–85.
79. Eger EI 2nd. Age, minimum alveolar anesthetic concentration, and minimum alveolar anesthetic concentration-awake. Anesth Analg 2001;93(4):947–53.
80. Nickalls RW, Mapleson WW. Age-related iso-MAC charts for isoflurane, sevoflurane and desflurane in man. Br J Anaesth 2003;91(2):170–4.
81. Lawrence VA, Cornell JE, Smetana GW, American College of Physicians. Strategies to reduce postoperative pulmonary complications after noncardiothoracic surgery: systematic review for the American College of Physicians. Ann Intern Med 2006;144(8):596–608.

82. Berg H, Roed J, Viby-Mogensen J, et al. Residual neuromuscular block is a risk factor for postoperative pulmonary complications. A prospective, randomised, and blinded study of postoperative pulmonary complications after atracurium, vecuronium and pancuronium. Acta Anaesthesiol Scand 1997;41(9): 1095–103.
83. Warner DO. Preventing postoperative pulmonary complications: the role of the anesthesiologist. Anesthesiology 2000;92(5):1467–72.
84. Hasukic S, Mesic D, Dizdarevic E, et al. Pulmonary function after laparoscopic and open cholecystectomy. Surg Endosc 2002;16(1):163–5.
85. Karayiannakis AJ, Makri GG, Mantzioka A, et al. Postoperative pulmonary function after laparoscopic and open cholecystectomy. Br J Anaesth 1996;77(4): 448–52.
86. Squadrone V, Coha M, Cerutti E, et al. Continuous positive airway pressure for treatment of postoperative hypoxemia: a randomized controlled trial. JAMA 2005;293(5):589–95.
87. Ferreyra GP, Baussano I, Squadrone V, et al. Continuous positive airway pressure for treatment of respiratory complications after abdominal surgery: a systematic review and meta-analysis. Ann Surg 2008;247(4):617–26.
88. Thompson LF. Failure to wean: exploring the influence of age-related pulmonary changes. Crit Care Nurs Clin North Am 1996;8(1):7–16.
89. Sloane PJ, Gee MH, Gottlieb JE, et al. A multicenter registry of patients with acute respiratory distress syndrome. Physiology and outcome. Am Rev Respir Dis 1992;146(2):419–26.
90. Terragni PP, Antonelli M, Fumagalli R, et al. Early vs late tracheotomy for prevention of pneumonia in mechanically ventilated adult ICU patients: a randomized controlled trial. JAMA 2010;303(15):1483–9.
91. Guimaraes MM, El Dib R, Smith AF, et al. Incentive spirometry for prevention of postoperative pulmonary complications in upper abdominal surgery. Cochrane Database Syst Rev 2009;(3):CD006058.
92. Carvalho CR, Paisani DM, Lunardi AC. Incentive spirometry in major surgeries: a systematic review. Rev Bras Fisioter 2011;15(5):343–50.
93. Overend TJ, Anderson CM, Lucy SD, et al. The effect of incentive spirometry on postoperative pulmonary complications: a systematic review. Chest 2001; 120(3):971–8.
94. Pasquina P, Tramer MR, Granier JM, et al. Respiratory physiotherapy to prevent pulmonary complications after abdominal surgery: a systematic review. Chest 2006;130(6):1887–99.
95. Craig DB, Wahba WM, Don HF, et al. "Closing volume" and its relationship to gas exchange in seated and supine positions. J Appl Physiol (1985) 1971;31(5): 717–21.
96. Shafer SL. The pharmacology of anesthetic drugs in elderly patients. Anesthesiol Clin North America 2000;18(1):1–29, v.
97. Walder B, Schafer M, Henzi I, et al. Efficacy and safety of patient-controlled opioid analgesia for acute postoperative pain. A quantitative systematic review. Acta Anaesthesiol Scand 2001;45(7):795–804.
98. Mann C, Pouzeratte Y, Boccara G, et al. Comparison of intravenous or epidural patient-controlled analgesia in the elderly after major abdominal surgery. Anesthesiology 2000;92(2):433–41.
99. Nordquist D, Halaszynski TM. Perioperative multimodal anesthesia using regional techniques in the aging surgical patient. Pain Res Treat 2014;2014: 902174.

100. Fong HK, Sands LP, Leung JM. The role of postoperative analgesia in delirium and cognitive decline in elderly patients: a systematic review. Anesth Analg 2006;102(4):1255–66.
101. Popping DM, Elia N, Marret E, et al. Protective effects of epidural analgesia on pulmonary complications after abdominal and thoracic surgery: a meta-analysis. Arch Surg 2008;143(10):990–9 [discussion: 1000].
102. Davies RG, Myles PS, Graham JM. A comparison of the analgesic efficacy and side-effects of paravertebral vs epidural blockade for thoracotomy–a systematic review and meta-analysis of randomized trials. Br J Anaesth 2006; 96(4):418–26.
103. Joshi GP, Bonnet F, Shah R, et al. A systematic review of randomized trials evaluating regional techniques for postthoracotomy analgesia. Anesth Analg 2008; 107(3):1026–40.
104. Zhang H, Lu Y, Liu M, et al. Strategies for prevention of postoperative delirium: a systematic review and meta-analysis of randomized trials. Critical 2013;17(2):R47.
105. Sieber FE, Mears S, Lee H, et al. Postoperative opioid consumption and its relationship to cognitive function in older adults with hip fracture. J Am Geriatr Soc 2011;59(12):2256–62.
106. Brouquet A, Cudennec T, Benoist S, et al. Impaired mobility, ASA status and administration of tramadol are risk factors for postoperative delirium in patients aged 75 years or more after major abdominal surgery. Ann Surg 2010;251(4): 759–65.
107. Teslyar P, Stock VM, Wilk CM, et al. Prophylaxis with antipsychotic medication reduces the risk of post-operative delirium in elderly patients: a meta-analysis. Psychosomatics 2013;54(2):124–31.

Effect of Aging on Renal Function Plus Monitoring and Support

 CrossMark

Anthony J. Baldea, MD

KEYWORDS

• Elderly patients • Aging kidney • Acute kidney injury • Renal replacement therapy

KEY POINTS

- There are several histologic changes in the aging kidney that occur as a patient grows older, including renovascular changes, tubulointerstitial fibrosis, glomerulosclerosis, and loss of nephrons.
- The structural changes of the aging kidney are accompanied by physiologic alterations in renal function, with a decreased ability of autoregulation of renal blood flow, diminished capacity to maintain water and electrolyte homeostasis, and heightened sensitivity to changes in renal blood flow.
- The net effects of the anatomic changes and alterations in renal physiology in the elderly patient lead to an increased susceptibility toward developing hypovolemia.
- Acute kidney injury (AKI) is common in hospitalized elderly patients, and leads to substantial morbidity and mortality; although the causes of AKI in the elderly are the same as in the general population, the distribution of the causes is slightly shifted.
- No specific therapy exists for treatment of the elderly patient with AKI; treatment is mainly supportive and should include the full spectrum of therapies offered to younger patients, including renal replacement therapy.

INTRODUCTION

Because of advances in medical therapy, the elderly represent the fastest growing segment of the general population. It is projected that, in the United States and Western Europe alone, there will be an increase in individuals older than 60 years from 231 million in 2000 to approximately 400 million by 2050.[1] To care for this rapidly increasing portion of the population, it is essential for clinicians to comprehend the effects that aging has on normal physiology, and the accompanying clinical consequences that these physiologic alterations can have when these elderly patients are

Disclosure: the author has nothing to disclose.
Division of Trauma, Critical Care and Burns, Loyola University Medical Center, 2160 South First Avenue, EMS Building, Room 3279, Maywood, IL 60153, USA
E-mail address: abaldea@lumc.edu

confronted with illness or injury. As patients age, several accompanying histologic alterations in renal functioning occur. The onset of these architectural and anatomic changes leads to subsequent physiologic perturbations, which can affect the care and prognosis of the elderly patient. Geriatric patients with chronic kidney disease (CKD) are particularly predisposed toward the development of acute kidney injury (AKI) and its adverse clinical sequelae. Understanding the mechanisms by which aging renal function deteriorates can lead to a better comprehension of how clinicians should approach the care of the injured or critically ill elderly patient.

THE EFFECTS OF AGING ON RENAL STRUCTURE

Several structural changes occur in the aging kidney, starting with histologic alterations in the renal vasculature (**Box 1**). Microangiopathic examination shows arteriolar deposition of subendothelial collagen fibers and hyaline, in addition to proliferation of elastic tissue, the sum of which leads to intimal thickening of both the afferent and efferent renal arterioles. These histologic changes are often associated with the development of atherosclerosis and atrophy of the smooth muscular media.[2] There is also a decreased ability in the capacity of the aging kidney to preserve the autonomic renal vascular reflex, which is termed renovascular dysautonomy; this diminished ability to maintain homeostasis can modify the ability to preserve renal function in both hypotensive and hypertensive states. Expansion of the mesangial matrix in the aging kidney induces destruction and extirpation of juxtamedullary nephrons, producing direct configurations and communication between the afferent and efferent arterioles. This structural process gives rise to a glomerular circulation, in which normal renal blood flow is compromised; the average decrease in renal blood flow is approximately 10% per decade starting at age 40 years.[3]

Box 1
Histologic changes in the aging kidney

Renal vasculature
- Subendothelial deposition of collagen fibers and hyaline in arterioles
- Proliferation of elastic tissue
- Atherosclerosis
- Smooth muscular medial atrophy

Mesangial matrix expansion

Aglomerular circulation

Glomerulosclerosis

Renal tubular atrophy, fibrosis and loss

Interstitial fibrosis

Decreased availability of functional sodium-potassium-chloride transporters

Nuclear changes
- Decreased tubular cell proliferation
- Increased susceptibility to apoptosis
- Telomere shortening
- Aberrant DNA methylation

Structural distortions within the functioning renal parenchyma also occur during the senescence process. Glomerular tissue is slowly replaced by fibrous tissue over time, leading toward the development of glomerulosclerosis, and is manifested by the loss of 30% to 50% of cortical glomeruli by age 70 years.[3] The renal tubules themselves are also affected over time, with the onset of tubular atrophy, decreased tubular number and length, fatty degeneration, and fibrosis. These histologic changes lead to tubular frailty, in which the tubule is less tolerant of nephrotoxic or hypoxic injury. The renal tubular countercurrent exchange established by the loops of Henle (and the surrounding vasa recta) is likewise affected over time, leading to the evolution of renal medullary hypotonicity. The net effect of this medullary hypotonicity is a decreased response to antidiuretic hormone and subsequent reduction in water reabsorption. Inflammatory cell accumulation and fibroblast deposition in the interstitial matrix precipitate interstitial fibrosis.[4,5] Furthermore, the nuclear ramifications of aging and cellular senescence include decreased tubular cell proliferation, increased susceptibility to apoptosis, telomere shortening, and aberrant DNA methylation, leading to an average loss of approximately 4500 nephrons per kidney per year during the aging process. There is an associated decrease in renal mass with aging, with a loss of approximately 25% to 30% by age 80 years.[6]

THE EFFECTS OF AGING ON RENAL PHYSIOLOGY AND THE RESULTANT CLINICAL CONSEQUENCES

The physiologic sequelae of these histologic alterations in renal structure in the aging kidney often start after the third decade of life (**Box 2**). Even healthy elderly individuals experience a progressive deterioration of glomerular filtration rate (GFR) as they age, with an average decrease of 0.8 to 1.0 mL/min/1.73 m^2 per year.[2,3] The usual effects of aging include senile sarcopenia, with a degenerative loss of skeletal muscle at a rate of approximately 0.5% to 1.0% loss per year after age 25 years; this sarcopenia is accompanied by a resultant decrease in creatinine production. As a result, progressive deterioration in the GFR in the aging kidney is not necessarily associated with a concomitant increase in the serum creatinine level.

Box 2
Physiologic changes in the elderly patient
Renovascular dysautonomy
Renal medullary hypotonicity
Sarcopenia
Tubular frailty
Decreased distal tubular sodium reabsorption
Blunted response to arginine vasopressin
Reduced free water clearance
Inability to maximally concentrate urine
Decreased production of vasodilatory prostaglandins
Decreased aldosterone levels
Relative tubular resistance to aldosterone
Decreased ability to renally excrete potassium
Diminished tubular urea reabsorption

The ability to maintain electrolyte and water homeostasis also diminishes with aging. Handling of sodium is particularly affected, with a blunted response to large sodium loads, and a decreased ability to compensate for sodium depletion. The functional capacity of the thick ascending loop of Henle to resorb sodium is drastically different between the kidneys of young individuals and aging patients, believed to be secondary to a decreased availability of functional sodium-potassium-chloride transporters; approximately 85% of elderly patients show reduced sodium reabsorption in this region.[7] Proximal sodium reabsorption is not likewise universally affected. In elderly patients, a decrease in thirst regulation and a blunted response of arginine vasopressin release in hypovolemic states result in alterations in water equilibrium. A 60% reduction in the free water clearance in the thick ascending loop of Henle also occurs with age. As a result of all these changes, the development of chronic hyponatremia secondary to senile sodium leakage and water disequilibrium is common in geriatric patients. Furthermore, renal medullary hypotonicity causes a reduced capacity to maximally concentrate urine, further predisposing elderly patients toward the development of dehydration.[2,8]

Normal efferent arteriolar tone is maintained by a balance between the vasoconstrictive effects of the renin-angiotensin-aldosterone axis and the vasodilatory effects of secreted prostaglandins. The aging kidney has a decreased production of vasodilatory prostaglandins, leading to an altered balance in arteriolar tone regulation, and an ensuing enhanced response to vasoconstrictive stimuli.[9,10] The net effect of these changes leads to an increased susceptibility to diminished renal blood flow during times of stress, which can result from hypovolemia, changes in cardiac output or medication effects (ie, nonsteroidal antiinflammatory drugs [NSAIDs]).

The structural changes in the aging kidney, in addition to decreased aldosterone levels and a relative resistance to aldosterone at the tubular level in the elderly patient, impair the ability of the aging kidney to appropriately secrete potassium, making older patients more prone to developing hyperkalemia. Also, an age-related reduction in the functioning number of urea channels in the distal tubules leads to a decreased capacity of urea reabsorption; this alteration in urea handling may contribute to the onset of nocturia in older patients (secondary to urea osmotic diuresis).

DEFINITION AND EPIDEMIOLOGY OF ACUTE KIDNEY INJURY IN THE ELDERLY

The consensus definition of AKI has undergone several modifications in recent years, to more accurately define and report perturbations in renal physiology. The Acute Dialysis Quality Insurance group[11] proposed the 5-stage RIFLE (risk, injury, failure, loss, end-stage renal disease [ESRD]) criteria in 2004 in an attempt to achieve this universal diagnostic and risk stratification classification. A 2007 modification of this classification scheme by the Acute Kidney Injury Network[12] added further specifications to the RIFLE criteria, and proposed 3 different stages for AKI from the RIFLE criteria: stage 1 (risk), stage 2 (injury), and stage 3 (failure). The loss and ESRD components were eliminated as stages, in an attempt to separate stages of disease from outcomes. Subsequent clinical practice guidelines released by the Kidney Disease/ Improving Global Outcomes (KDIGO) group in 2012 included additional modifications to the definition of AKI.[13] These most recent criteria use changes in serum creatinine and urine output. Per this classification scheme, AKI is defined as one of the following: an absolute increase in the serum creatinine level by 0.3 mg/dL or more within 48 hours, a relative increase in serum creatinine level by 1.5 or more times the baseline level, or a decrease in the urinary output of less than 0.5 mL/kg/h for a period of 6 hours.

Regardless of how it is defined, AKI is more prevalent as patients age, with a clear age-dependent relationship consistently shown between AKI and older age. The incidence of AKI in elderly hospitalized patients in the United States was 3.1% in 2000[14]; more recent subsequent studies have reported an even higher incidence. Based on numerous reports, the relative risk of AKI in the elderly compared with younger patients has been reported to be from a 3.5-fold to 10- fold increased risk. The incidence of AKI in elderly patients admitted to the intensive care unit (ICU) is even higher; data from the multicenter 2011 NEFROINT study[15] (RIFLE-based data collection/management system applied to a prospective cohort multicenter Italian study on the epidemiology of acute kidney injury in the intensive care unit) showed that 42.7% of 576 studied patients (median age 67 years) were diagnosed with AKI within 24 hours of admission to the ICU, and AKI developed in an additional 23% later in their hospital course.

RISK FACTORS FOR ACUTE KIDNEY INJURY IN THE ELDERLY

Several risk factors for AKI in the elderly have been reported in the literature; these risk factors can be broken down into underlying comorbidities, exposure to potentially nephrotoxic medications, and genetic factors. In a 2008 study by Hsu and colleagues[16] of 1764 hospitalized patients in the Kaiser Permanente system in Northern California, elderly patients with preexisting diabetes mellitus (DM), hypertension, and proteinuria were determined to be independent risk factors for developing AKI during hospitalization. A 2011 study from Huang and colleagues[17] reported that increasing severity of preoperative proteinuria correlated with the development of AKI as well as with the need for RRT in patients undergoing coronary artery bypass grafting surgery.

CKD, defined as an estimated GFR (eGFR) less than 60 mL/min/1.73 m^2, is another independent risk factor for AKI. Elderly patients with an eGFR between 45 and 59 mL/min/1.73 m^2 have approximately 2 times the risk of AKI compared with matched cohorts with an eGFR of 60 mL/min/1.73 m^2 or greater. In patients with baseline eGFR less than 60 mL/min/1.73 m^2, the presence of DM further augments the risk for AKI. Furthermore, as the eGFR decreases, the risk for AKI increases dramatically.[18] According to the 2008 study by Hsu and colleagues, patients with a baseline eGFR less than 15 mL/min/1.73 m^2 were particularly predisposed to developing AKI, with an adjusted odds ratio of AKI of 38.24 and 44.84 in the absence and presence of DM, respectively. Other studies have reported an increased risk of AKI in patients with atherosclerosis, congestive heart failure, or renovascular disease.

Elderly patients taking angiotensin-converting enzyme (ACE) inhibitors, angiotensin receptor blockers (ARB), or NSAIDs before their hospitalization also seem to be at an increased risk of developing AKI, secondary to the effects that those medications have on the autoregulatory ability of the aging kidney in times of stress and hemodynamic changes. Furthermore, it is surmised that elderly patients are particularly predisposed to AKI secondary to medication usage because of decreased body mass, altered medication clearance, and the long half-lives of certain medications (such as with NSAIDs). Within the ICU, the most frequent specific adverse drug reaction in the elderly is drug-induced AKI; common offending agents include aminoglycosides, ACE inhibitors, NSAIDs, vancomycin, amphotericin B, cyclosporine, and tacrolimus.

Recent research has suggested that a variety of genetic factors in certain cohorts of elderly patients may be involved in predisposing individuals to AKI, and also regulating the recovery of renal function. Proposed mechanisms affecting the development and recovery from AKI include the expression of specific microRNA, degree of telomere shortening, heme-oxygenase modulated autophagy, and chordin 1–regulated expression of bone morphogenic protein 7 in restoring tubular epithelium after injury.[19]

Further research in this area is needed to understand the clinical ramifications of genetic factors in the development of AKI, as well as to highlight potential areas for therapeutic mediation in this regard.

CAUSE OF ACUTE KIDNEY INJURY IN THE ELDERLY

Although the literature delineating the underlying cause of AKI in elderly patients is not robust, the available data suggest that approximately 35% of cases have prerenal causes, 40% have intrarenal (intrinsic) causes, and 25% are secondary to postrenal (obstructive) causes.[20] Although the typical causes of AKI in the elderly patient mirror those seen in the general population, the previously mentioned alterations in renal structure and physiology with aging lead to some potential differences in the distribution of cause.

Prerenal Acute Kidney Injury

Prerenal AKI in the elderly patient can be secondary to any underlying cause of decreased renal perfusion (**Box 3**). As in the general population, it is most commonly a result of volume depletion, which can be secondary to gastrointestinal losses (diarrhea, vomiting), renal losses (such as with diuretic use), or intravascular losses (third spacing from pancreatitis or after surgery, hemorrhage). For the reasons mentioned earlier, elderly patients are particularly prone to the development of dehydration during times of physiologic stress and have a decreased adaptive ability to maintain renal blood flow and GFR. Prerenal states can also develop from other causes of diminished effective arterial blood volume, which can transpire in patients with congestive heart failure, nephrotic syndrome, or cirrhosis. Profound hypercalcemia, often secondary to an underlying malignancy, can likewise lead to a state of volume depletion in the elderly patient. Diuretics are frequently prescribed medications in the elderly population and have been estimated to contribute to volume depletion in approximately 25% to 40% of the cases of prerenal AKI in elderly patients.[21] As mentioned earlier, ACE inhibitors, ARB, and NSAIDs all can alter renal hemodynamics and lead to a prerenal state.

Intrinsic Acute Kidney Injury

Intrinsic renal causes of AKI are caused by structural insults and damage to the kidney that endure after the implicating factor is withdrawn (**Box 4**). The most prevalent form

---

Box 3
Common causes of prerenal AKI in the elderly patient

Hypovolemia

- Gastrointestinal tract losses (diarrhea, vomiting)
- Inadequate oral intake
- Renal losses (diuretic medications, osmotic diuresis)
- Intravascular losses (hemorrhage, third spacing)

Diminished effective arterial volume

- Cirrhosis
- Congestive heart failure or valvular disease
- Nephrotic syndrome

Medication administration (NSAIDs, ACE inhibitors, ARB, calcineurin inhibitors)

Hypercalcemia

| Box 4 |
| Common causes of intrinsic AKI in the elderly patient |

Acute tubular necrosis

- Ischemia
- Sepsis
- Direct nephrotoxicity (medications, contrast-induced nephropathy)
- Prolonged volume depletion with delayed resuscitation

Acute interstitial nephritis

- Medications (penicillins, sulfonamides, proton-pump inhibitors, NSAIDs, cephalosporins)
- Infection
- Systemic collagen vascular disease

Vascular causes

- Atheroembolic disease
- Vasculitis
- Renal vein thrombosis
- Renal artery dissection

of intrinsic AKI in the elderly patient is from acute tubular necrosis (ATN), which can occur secondary to direct nephrotoxicity, ischemia, sepsis, and prolonged volume depletion with delayed resuscitation. Nephrotoxic agents implicated in the development of ATN in the elderly include aminoglycosides, amphotericin, and cisplatinum. Direct nephrotoxicity can also result from heme-pigment deposition and direct tubular injury, as is shown in rhabdomyolysis and hemolysis. Ischemic ATN is often identified in the elderly surgical patient, most commonly after cardiac and aortic procedures. Septic ATN results from endotoxemia-induced renal vasoconstriction and is the underlying cause of approximately one-third of cases of ATN in elderly patients.

As mentioned earlier, intrinsic AKI may result from contrast-induced nephropathy (CIN), particularly when high-volume or high-osmolar contrast is administered to a volume-depleted patient. Hospitalized elderly patients often are subjected to intravenous contrast media administration for both diagnostic studies (ie, contrast-enhanced computed tomography [CT] imaging) and therapeutic interventions (ie, coronary angiography). The available data suggest that elderly patients are at an increased risk of developing CIN compared with younger patients. A 2014 meta-analysis[22] of 22 studies on this topic reported an overall incidence of CIN in 13.6% of patients older than 65 years who were exposed to contrast administration. More specifically, there was a 12.4% incidence of CIN in the group of elderly patients receiving intravenous contrast, and a 15.5% incidence of CIN in those who were administered intracoronary contrast. When matching for comorbidities, a risk-adjusted analysis in this study showed that elderly patients were 2 times more likely to develop CIN than younger patients.

Another, perhaps underrecognized, cause of intrinsic AKI in the elderly patient is from acute interstitial nephritis (AIN), implicated in approximately 5% of cases.[3] The classic triad of presentation of AIN involves the development of rash, fever, and eosinophilia. AIN is usually related to infection, systemic collagen vascular diseases, or (most commonly) from adverse drug reactions; some common culprits of medications leading to AIN are sulfonamides, penicillin-based products, cephalosporins, proton-pump inhibitors, and NSAIDs. The usual onset of AIN secondary to hypersensitivity to medications is within 2 weeks of administration, although the timing varies dramatically, and it can develop up to several months after the initiation of NSAID use.

A variety of vascular causes can lead to intrinsic AKI in the elderly patient, most commonly from atheroembolic disease. Diffuse atherosclerosis leads to showering of cholesterol plaques into the microcirculation, eliciting a robust inflammatory response, which can subsequently occlude small vessels. The renal vasculature is a frequently involved location, because of the high rate of renal blood flow compared with other organs. Other vascular causes leading to intrinsic AKI include vasculitis, renal vein thrombosis, and renal artery dissection. Less common, nonvascular causes of intrinsic AKI include myeloma neuropathy and rapidly progressive glomerulonephritis.

Postrenal Acute Kidney Injury

Postrenal, or obstructive, causes of AKI are more common in the elderly than in younger patients. These causes can be further divided into upper urinary tract (obstruction occurring proximal to the bladder) and lower urinary tract (at the level of the bladder outlet or urethra). Upper urinary tract obstructive causes include previous radiation therapy, nephrolithiasis, and malignancy. Upper urinary tract obstruction may result in unilateral hydronephrosis and possibly renal colic, but does not necessarily result in AKI if the other kidney is able to compensate. AKI can occur from cases of bilateral upper urinary tract obstruction or unilateral obstruction in a solitary kidney. In contrast, lower urinary tract causes of obstruction have a greater propensity to affect the bilateral kidneys and lead to impairment in renal function. Obstruction at this level occurs most commonly from benign or malignant prostatic obstruction, but can also be secondary to bladder malignancy, retroperitoneal or pelvic malignancies, neurogenic causes, previous trauma with subsequent urethral stricture or blood clots causing a bladder outlet obstruction.

DIAGNOSIS AND MONITORING OF ACUTE KIDNEY INJURY

Although monitoring of the serum creatinine level is the most extensively used, studied, and validated marker for decreased GFR and development of AKI in the elderly patient, its correlation with AKI has some important limitations. The interpretation of serum creatinine level as a surrogate for GFR is dependent on the complex interaction between volume of distribution, renal elimination, and creatinine generation, all of which can be substantially altered in the elderly patient. Thus, monitoring relative (and not absolute) changes in the serum creatinine level, as per the KDIGO criteria, may be a more dependable marker of AKI in the elderly patient. Estimations of GFR in addition to monitoring of urinary output can also be useful adjuncts toward the early recognition of AKI in this distinct population. Several recent studies have evaluated the usefulness of novel biomarkers for the early diagnosis of AKI in critically ill elderly patients.[23–25] Urinary interleukin 18, cystatin C, and neutrophil-associated gelatinase-associated lipocalin have all shown promise as potential biomarkers as an early indication of acute renal dysfunction, although more work is still needed to validate their clinical usefulness.

Once the diagnosis of AKI has been made, the workup should start with a thorough history and physical examination to delineate if the cause is prerenal, intrinsic, or postrenal in nature. A history of dehydration, massive gastrointestinal tract fluid losses, or episodes of hypotension may indicate hypovolemia or ischemia. Physical examination findings and eliciting a full history can assist in identifying obstructive causes of AKI. Recent medication use should be thoroughly evaluated, in an attempt to identify and discontinue any potentially nephrotoxic agents. All medication doses should be adjusted to accommodate the change in renal function, and drugs that can cause further nephrotoxicity should be avoided if possible.

Urinalysis can alert the clinician as to the underlying cause of AKI. The presence of pigmented granular casts in the urine is a marker of tubular injury and is consistent with ATN. The finding of white blood cells in the urine and subnephrotic proteinuria may facilitate the diagnosis of AIN, particularly when there is an associated predominance of eosinophils; however, eosinophiluria is neither sensitive nor specific in establishing the diagnosis of AIN, and it also occurs in a variety of other disorders (including atheroembolic disease, cystitis, and prostatitis). Glomerulonephritis is suggested with the presence of dysmorphic red blood cell casts in the urine; definitive diagnosis should be confirmed by obtaining a kidney biopsy.

Checking urine electrolyte and creatinine levels can be used to calculate the fractional excretion of sodium (FeNa); a prerenal cause of AKI is typically associated with a low urine sodium level and a FeNa of less than 1%, whereas with intrinsic causes of AKI the FeNa is usually greater than 3%. In patients who have recently been administered diuretics, renal sodium absorption and excretion may be altered as a result, thus making the interpretation of the FeNa more challenging. In this patient population, measuring the fractional excretion of urea is preferred, with a calculated level less than 40% consistent with a prerenal cause.

The diagnosis of postrenal AKI is confirmed with the finding of urinary retention on bladder scan or with increased postvoid residual bladder volumes. Radiographic workup often starts with ultrasonography, which can show hydronephrosis and hydroureter. CT is often useful when ultrasonography is nondiagnostic, as can be seen in cases of early upper urinary tract obstruction.

PREVENTION AND TREATMENT OF ACUTE KIDNEY INJURY

Although there are no treatment measures specific to the elderly population once AKI has occurred, attempts should be focused on identifying elderly patients at risk for the development of AKI, and mitigating perturbations in renal function by modifying potentially reversible causes of AKI. Perhaps the most important principle toward prevention of AKI in these patients is understanding that increases in the serum creatinine level may not be the most reliable early indicator of AKI and should not be relied on as a sole measure of renal function. For those patients with underlying CKD, all medications should be appropriately dosed to prevent nephrotoxic adverse drug effects. As described earlier, elderly patients are particularly predisposed toward quickly developing hypovolemia, and thus, adequate volume resuscitation should be ensured, with the early use of invasive cardiac monitoring as necessary. Although there are no specific recommendations for preventing AKI in the elderly patients, the European Society of Intensive Care Medicine (ESICM) recommends maintaining a mean arterial pressure (MAP) greater than 60 mm Hg to maintain renal perfusion.[26] The goal blood pressure should be tailored to each individual patient, because a higher goal MAP may be beneficial in some patients with other comorbidities (ie, untreated hypertension). All elderly patients should be considered at increased risk for CIN, and adequate circulating volume status should be maintained before receiving contrast media. The role of bicarbonate supplementation and the administration of N-acetylcysteine are less clear in the prevention of CIN.

Although there is no consensus on which particular intravenous fluid should be administered for correction of intravascular volume depletion in the elderly patient, the mainstay of therapy is typically an isotonic crystalloid fluid. Some recent studies have reported a correlation between administration of high-molecular-weight hydrox-yethylstarch solutions and an increased risk of developing AKI. Accordingly, the 2010 guidelines from the ESICM recommend against the use of colloids during the initial resuscitation of patients with septic shock or hypovolemia.[26] The goal of volume resuscitation should be to restore euvolemia, with the cognizance that overresuscita-tion of the elderly patient can lead to a variety of adverse sequelae, including pul-monary edema, peripheral edema, anasarca, worsening AKI, and abdominal compartment syndrome. The clinician should be vigilant about monitoring for the un-toward clinical manifestations of overresuscitation, and use clinical end points to assist in guiding a judicious volume resuscitation, using urinary output and invasive cardiovascular monitoring as necessary to tailor a well-guided resuscitation.

Akin to the population in general, there are no specific therapies for AKI in elderly patients once the renal insult has occurred. Management strategies focus on limiting the extent of injury and preserving as much renal function as possible. The mainstays of support for elderly patients with AKI include sustaining adequate renal blood flow, with appropriate hemodynamic monitoring as necessary.

The literature does not report inferior outcomes after renal replacement therapy (RRT) in the elderly when compared with younger patients with the same severity of illness; thus, general supportive measures for a patient with AKI requiring RRT should not be withheld from a patient based solely on age. In general, the literature supports the notion that RRT is effective, well tolerated, and safe in the elderly population.[1,27,28] Thus, the same indications for RRT that would be offered to younger patients should be offered to the elderly. Although no large, prospective studies have specifically addressed whether a particular modality or intensity of RRT is superior in the treatment of elderly patients requiring RRT after AKI, there are no overwhelming data in the liter-ature supporting one modality over another in the general population. The choice of modality and intensity of RRT depends on a full evaluation of the elderly patient's abil-ity to tolerate the various modes of RRT, because of the patient's underlying comor-bidities, intravascular volume status, and alterations in cardiovascular physiology.

OUTCOMES AFTER ACUTE KIDNEY INJURY

Using data from both experimental animal models as well as from human studies, the pathophysiologic sequelae of AKI are becoming more recognized. Within several days to weeks after an episode of AKI, there is a vigorous inflammatory response within the healing kidney, often leading to tubulointerstitial fibrosis, architectural remodeling, and subsequent changes in renal physiology. The fibrotic response is multifactorial in cause: structural and physiologic manifestations mediated by an upregulation of the genes responsible for inflammation, direct damage to the renal microvasculature, the consequences of ischemia-reperfusion injury, and alterations in sensitivity to the renin-angiotensin-aldosterone pathway.[18] This response seems to be accentuated in the aging kidney. Accordingly, elderly patients are at an increased risk for failure of recovery of kidney function after AKI. A 2008 meta-analysis of 17 studies[29] reported that the rate of recovery of kidney function after AKI was 68.7% in elderly patients compared with 74% in those younger than 65 years (pooled relative risk, 1.28; P<.05).

Mortality

The in-house mortality for elderly patients who experience AKI during their hospitali-zation ranges in the literature from 15% to 40%.[20] AKI also seems to be an important predictor of long-term mortality in the elderly population: results from the 2009 Medi-care study[14] showed that the 2-year mortality in elderly hospital survivors after an episode of AKI was 57.7%, compared with a 2-year mortality of 28.2% of patients without AKI. The 2-year mortality was 64.3% in the subset of discharged elderly patients with AKI who had underlying CKD and was 54.3% in those with AKI but without CKD. The effect of AKI on long-term mortality is shown by contrasting this mortality with the overall 37.9% 2-year mortality in discharged patients (from the same database) with CKD but without AKI. The relative risk for death within certain age cohorts in the elderly does not seem to be substantially different; a multicenter prospective study of 725 patients with AKI was performed by the Madrid Acute Renal Failure Study Group,[30] and did not show a statistically significant difference in mortality after AKI for patients aged 65 to 79 years and those older than 80 years.

Progression to Chronic Kidney Disease and End-Stage Renal Disease

Although the traditional belief underlying AKI was that it was a reversible condition, with no long-term sequelae in hospital survivors who recover kidney function, recent studies have shown that all patients with AKI, including the elderly, are at an increased risk for subsequently developing CKD or ESRD. A longitudinal study with 10-year follow-up of 187 patients surviving AKI[31] reported with regression analysis that age, comorbidities, and renal function at discharge were all independent predictors of long-term functional outcome after AKI in hospital survivors.

The long-term recovery of renal function after AKI in elderly patients is at least partially predicated on the patient's underlying renal function before sustaining the AKI. In a 2009 retrospective analysis of more than 233,000 Medicare beneficiaries,[14] the 2-year progression to ESRD was examined in elderly patients who were discharged with a diagnosis of AKI during their hospitalization. Compared with epidemiologically similar and morbidity-adjusted cohorts without any kidney disease, there was a hazard ratio of 41.2 of developing ESRD in patients with CKD and AKI, with an overall 14.29% likelihood of initiating RRT within 2 years of hospital discharge. In patients with AKI and without previous CKD, the hazard ratio of developing ESRD was 13.0, with a 2-year probability of 6.96% of initiating RRT. Within this same study, the 2-year risk of developing CKD in those patients hospitalized with AKI was 72.1%. Other studies have reported that the risk for progression to ESRD is also related to the degree of AKI, with a higher incidence of progression to ESRD seen in elderly patients with severe AKI compared with those with mild AKI.

SUMMARY

Elderly patients comprise an ever-increasing segment of the population. There are several anatomic changes and physiologic alterations that occur in the aging kidney, which in sum account for the elderly patient's modified ability to maintain renal function in times of stress. Keeping these structural and physiologic changes in mind is essential for the early recognition of AKI and improving outcomes in hospitalized elderly patients. There are no specific diagnostic methods or treatment modalities that are unique in the care of the elderly patient with AKI. Therapy is mainly supportive, and the full spectrum of treatment options, including RRT, should not be withheld from a patient based solely on age. More studies need to be performed to determine the optimal timing, intensity, and modality of RRT in the elderly population.

REFERENCES

1. Van Den Noortgate N, Mouton V, Lamot C, et al. Outcome in a post-cardiac surgery population with acute renal failure requiring dialysis: does age make a difference? Nephrol Dial Transplant 2003;18(4):732-6.

2. Musso CG, Oreopoulos DG. Aging and physiological changes of the kidneys including changes in glomerular filtration rate. Nephron Physiol 2011;119(Suppl 1):p1–5.

3. Abdel-Kader K, Palevsky PM. Acute kidney injury in the elderly. Clin Geriatr Med 2009;25(3):331–58.

4. Silva FG. The ageing kidney: a review. I. Int Urol Nephrol 2005;37:185–205.

5. Silva FG. The ageing kidney: a review. II. Int Urol Nephrol 2005;37:419–32.

6. Lindeman RD. Overview: renal physiology and pathophysiology of aging. Am J Kidney Dis 1990;16(4):275–82.

7. Musso CG. Geriatric nephrology and the 'nephrogeriatric giants'. Int Urol Nephrol 2002;34:255–6.

8. Pascual J, Liano F, Ortuno J, et al. The elderly patient with acute renal failure. J Am Soc Nephrol 1995;6(2):144–53.

9. Castellani S, Ungar A, Cantini C, et al. Excessive vasoconstriction after stress by the aging kidney: inadequate prostaglandin modulation of increased endothelin activity. J Lab Clin Med 1998;132(3):186–94.

10. Crane MG, Harris JJ. Effect of aging on renin activity and aldosterone excretion. J Lab Clin Med 1976;87(6):947–59.

11. Bellomo R, Ronco C, Kellum JA, et al, Acute Dialysis Quality Initiative workgroup. Acute renal failure–definition, outcome measures, animal models, fluid therapy and information technology needs: the Second International Consensus Conference of the Acute Dialysis Quality Initiative (ADQI) Group. Crit Care 2004;8(4): R204–12.

12. Mehta RL, Kellum JA, Shah SV, et al, Acute Kidney Injury Network. Acute Kidney Injury Network: report of an initiative to improve outcomes in acute kidney injury. Crit Care 2007;11(2):R31.

13. Kidney Disease: Improving Global Outcomes (KDIGO) Acute Kidney Injury Work Group. KDIGO Clinical Practice Guideline for acute kidney injury. Kidney Int Suppl 2012;2:1–138.

14. Ishani A, Xue JL, Himmelfarb J, et al. Acute kidney injury increases risk of ESRD among elderly. J Am Soc Nephrol 2009;20(1):223–8.

15. Garzotto F, Piccinni P, Cruz D, et al, NEFROINT Investigation Group. RIFLE-based data collection/management system applied to a prospective cohort multicenter Italian study on the epidemiology of acute kidney injury in the intensive care unit. Blood Purif 2011;31(1–3):159–71.

16. Hsu CY, Ordoñez JD, Chertow GM, et al. The risk of acute renal failure in patients with chronic kidney disease. Kidney Int 2008;74(1):101–7.

17. Huang TM, Wu VC, Young GH, et al, National Taiwan University Hospital Study Group of Acute Renal Failure. Preoperative proteinuria predicts adverse renal outcomes after coronary artery bypass grafting. J Am Soc Nephrol 2011;22(1): 156–63.

18. Coca SG, Cho KC, Hsu CY. Acute kidney injury in the elderly: predisposition to chronic kidney disease and vice versa. Nephron Clin Pract 2011;119(Suppl 1): c19–24.

19. Del Giudice A, Piemontese M, Valente G, et al. Acute kidney injury in the elderly: epidemiology, risk factors and outcomes. J Nephrol Therapeut 2012;2:129.

20. Coca SG. Acute kidney injury in elderly persons. Am J Kidney Dis 2010;56(1): 122–31.

21. Van Kraaij DJ, Jansen RW, Gribnau FW, et al. Diuretic therapy in elderly heart failure patients with and without left ventricular systolic dysfunction. Drugs Aging 2000;16(4):289–300.

22. Song W, Zhang T, Pu J, et al. Incidence and risk of developing contrast-induced acute kidney injury following intravascular contrast administration in elderly patients. Clin Interv Aging 2014;9:85–93.
23. Herget-Rosenthal S, Marggraf G, Husing J, et al. Early detection of acute renal failure by serum cystatin C. Kidney Int 2004;66(3):1115–22.
24. Han WK, Waikar SS, Johnson A, et al. Urinary biomarkers in the early diagnosis of acute kidney injury. Kidney Int 2008;73(7):863–9.
25. Parikh CR, Mishra J, Thiessen-Philbrook H, et al. Urinary IL-18 is an early predictive biomarker of acute kidney injury after cardiac surgery. Kidney Int 2006;70(1):199–203.
26. Joannidis M, Druml W, Forni LG, et al, Critical Care Nephrology Working Group of the European Society of Intensive Care Medicine. Prevention of acute kidney injury and protection of renal function in the intensive care unit. Expert opinion of the Working Group for Nephrology, ESICM. Intensive Care Med 2010;36(3):392–411.
27. Akposso K, Hertig A, Couprie R, et al. Acute renal failure in patients over 80 years old: 25 years' experience. Intensive Care Med 2000;26:400–6.
28. Bonello MP, Ricci Z, Zamperetti N, et al. Critical care nephrology. In: Ronco CB, Kellum JA, editors. Acute renal failure in the elderly critically ill patient. Philadelphia: Saunders Elsevier; 2008. p. 1675–80.
29. Schmitt R, Coca S, Kanbay M, et al. Recovery of kidney function after acute kidney injury in the elderly: a systematic review and meta-analysis. Am J Kidney Dis 2008;52(2):262–71.
30. Pascual J, Liano F. Causes and prognosis of acute renal failure in the very old. Madrid Acute Renal Failure Study Group. J Am Geriatr Soc 1998;46(6):721–5.
31. Ponte B, Felipe C, Muriel A, et al. Long-term functional evolution after an acute kidney injury: a 10-year study. Nephrol Dial Transplant 2008;23(12):3859–66.

Management of the Gastrointestinal Tract and Nutrition in the Geriatric Surgical Patient

Eden Nohra, MD, Grant V. Bochicchio, MD, MPH*

KEYWORDS

• Geriatric patient • Malnutrition • Nutrition • Surgery

KEY POINTS

- Elderly people experience physiologic changes in the gut and in every organ system, which predisposes them to impaired nutrition and associated increased risk factors.
- When the normal processes of aging is compounded by illness, the propensity to cause a pathologic state of malnutrition increases.
- Surgical nutrition support in the critical care setting aims to identify those at nutritional risk and to support nutritional needs in the direction of recovery; new evidence has arisen for use of certain nutrients as therapeutic agents because they are thought to contribute to the healing process and may be conditionally deficient in stress related to disease processes.
- It is important that health care providers follow evidenced-based recommendations for the provision of adequate nutrients and address the individual needs of every patient.

INTRODUCTION

Increased age leads to the loss of cells in the myenteric plexus[1] and decreased gastric emptying, possibly associated with reduced nitric oxide concentrations.[1] Satiety is affected by a reduction in the endogenous-opioid–mediated feeding drive and by altered neurotransmitter signaling in brain hunger and satiety centers.[1] There is an enhanced secretion of cholecystokinin that inhibits gastric emptying and increases satiety.[1] The functions of ghrelin and glucagonlike peptide are also modified.[1] Slowing of gastric emptying prolongs satiety.[2] Because of the delay in gastric emptying associated with normal aging, elderly patients often are recommended liquid diets that are high in calories and protein.[1] Therefore, the changes in appetite and satiety are

Washington University in St. Louis School of Medicine, St Louis, MO, USA
* Corresponding author. Department of Surgery, Washington University School of Medicine, 660 South Euclid Avenue, CB 8109, St Louis, MO 63110.
E-mail address: bochicchiog@wudosis.wustl.edu

Surg Clin N Am 95 (2015) 85–101
http://dx.doi.org/10.1016/j.suc.2014.09.005
0039-6109/15/$ – see front matter © 2015 Elsevier Inc. All rights reserved.

surgical.theclinics.com

multiple and include both central and peripheral factors that are impacted by aging, and many of these changes continue to be poorly understood.[2]

Because of the above factors, age is considered a nonmodifiable risk factor involving surgical outcome. This statement is modulated by the effect of physiologic age versus chronologic age,[3] which is often expressed in clinical practice as the perceived condition of the patient with respect to what the clinician would expect for their specific biological age. Objective measures exist for biological age, such as the concept of frailty,[4] which has been defined recently as the presence of 4 of 6 of the following factors associated with the prediction of 6-month mortality: Mini-Cog score of 3 or less, albumin level of 3.3 mg/dL or less, more than 1 fall in the last 6 months, hematocrit level less than 35%, dependency with at least one activity of daily living, and the presence of at least 3 comorbidities.[5] Frailty assessment is currently recommended in the routine preoperative assessment of the elderly patient and has been associated with an increased surgical risk among several procedures and in diverse prospective cohorts.[6–8]

It is important to understand the uniqueness of the aging patient to achieve the best surgical outcome by applying necessary screening criteria and using risk-modifying interventions to address their special perioperative needs. The elderly are a segment of the population significantly increasing in numbers. The US Census Bureau estimates that old-age dependency will approach youth dependency in 2030 and will actually surpass it in 2060.[9] The "baby boomers" are currently 50 to 65 years of age and with the current life expectancy will cause a significantly larger portion of the population to be elderly.[9] The number of elderly patients in the United States is expected to double in the next 25 years.[10]

The nutritional status of the elderly surgical patient has been found to be of paramount importance in the prediction of surgical risk.[8] Furthermore, nutritional interventions are purported to alter this risk when applied appropriately.[8] In addition, the postoperative elderly individual is at a greater risk of malnutrition development and subsequent health and quality of life deterioration than a younger person.[11] This review discusses the importance of optimizing the outcome of the geriatric surgical patient through proper nutritional assessment and delivery of adequate nutrition via the gastrointestinal tract.

BACKGROUND

It is estimated that more than 50% of surgical procedures are performed on individuals older than 65 years and that one-half of all individuals older than 65 will require some type of operative procedure.[12] In 2010, more than one-third of all surgical operations were performed on patients 65 years of age and older.[13] As noted above, the number of elderly individuals is steadily increasing, and the population census estimates that more than 20% of individuals in the United States will be elderly by 2025.[9]

Because the number of elderly patients is increasing and the nutrition aspect of their care is likely a modifiable risk factor for improved outcome, it is important for medical providers to be well versed in identifying potential or existing nutritional problems in their patient. In addition, health care providers must be skilled at appropriately identifying risk factors for malnutrition and creating care plans to implement appropriate nutritional support and treatment proactively.

Malnutrition has been associated with increased postoperative complications,[14–16] perioperative mortality,[17,18] increased hospital length of stay,[17] decreased longevity,[11] and quality of life[11] in elderly patients with various disease conditions. Sadly, the prevalence of malnutrition in hospital and nursing home settings has been reported to be more than 40% to 50%.[19] It is, therefore, not uncommon for elderly patients to present for surgical consultation with some degree of malnutrition or cachexia.[8,20] Thus, it is imperative for the preoperative planning and surgical treatment plan to involve an overall nutritional assessment.[8] If the patient is severely malnourished, the decision to proceed with surgery may need to be delayed, as the risks of an adverse outcome may outweigh the benefits of surgical intervention.[8]

RISK FACTORS FOR MALNUTRITION IN THE ELDERLY

Medical or surgical illness impairing the function of the gastrointestinal tract is clearly a pathologic state causing a predisposition to malnutrition. Physical factors limiting eating ability[21] or interest in food may become pathologic states predisposing one to malnutrition. Such factors include poor dentition, swallowing dysfunction, poor vision,[21] and a weakened ability to secure or prepare food.[22] Social isolation may itself be a disease state because elderly individuals are inclined to eat less when they eat alone. Poor economic conditions lead to malnutrition because of food insecurity.[23] If an elderly person needs assistance with activities of daily living and help is not available, the individual will also be predisposed to malnutrition. Bereavement in the elderly may be a pathologic state because some elderly individuals may not recover fast enough after loss of a loved one without accruing long-term decline in their level of functioning.

Other psychological or pathologic diseases more common in the elderly are often associated with malnutrition states. For example, elderly individuals are predisposed to depression,[1] and the presentation may be subtle and missed by routine general assessment. Depression often leads to less eating and to malnourishment.[1] Dementia has been associated with malnourishment, although it is unclear whether malnourishment most often leads to decline in mental capacity or whether the lack of nourishment is a manifestation of dementia.[1]

Since the risks of neoplasia increases with age, a greater proportion of the elderly population has a neoplastic disease.[8] The cancer site itself (eg, gastric, esophageal) is associated with specific challenges to nutrition. Both surgical patients and patients receiving chemotherapy or radiotherapy may have better outcome when well nourished.[8] Patients who have undergone surgery for their disease are at greater risk for complications when they are malnourished and are at increased risk to remain malnourished postoperatively. The gastrointestinal system may be compromised by a surgical site complication and may have altered gastrointestinal physiology because of either their pre-existing gastric motility issues related to their age or a newly altered anatomy.

Biological Changes of the Gastrointestinal Tract

Age-related changes in the gastrointestinal tract are often impacted by concomitant pathologic factors or disease processes such as diabetes, pancreatitis, liver disease, and malignancy.[24] It may be difficult to discern whether the gastrointestinal dysfunction is the result of their aging or disease.

Dysphagia, gastrointestinal reflux, and constipation often are a result of neurodegeneration of the aging enteric nervous system.[24,25] In rodent studies, caloric reduction is found to prevent neuronal loss, proposing that diet alone may influence the aging gut.[24,26] Esophageal and gastric motility are impacted as a result of the reduction of neurons in the mesenteric plexus in older people[24,27]; however, the small intestine seems to be unaffected.[24,28] As we age, signal transduction pathways and cellular mechanisms that control smooth muscle contraction can influence the colonic motility, which may lead to constipation.[24,29]

A reduction in gastric acid secretions occurs with increasing age.[24] Chronic gastritis leads to hypochlorhydria and, as a consequence, proton pump inhibitors are frequently used for prolonged periods in older people, which causes suppressed acid secretion.[24] This decline in acid secretion predisposes the gut to small bowel bacterial overgrowth.[24,30] Bacterial overgrowth has been associated with weight loss and reduced intake of micronutrients.[24,31]

Structural changes of the pancreas are evident with the aging process.[24,32] Chymotrypsin and bicarbonate concentration in pancreatic juice have all been found to decrease with aging.[24,33] Others have reported that there is little evidence of reduced pancreatic secretion with age-independent factors such as disease and drugs.[24,34] With age, the liver decreases in size and blood flow, but microscopic changes seem to be subtle.[24,35] Aging mice studies have found that changes in the expression of genes in the liver are involved in inflammation, cellular stress, and fibrosis.[24,36] Limiting calories in mice seemed to reverse age-related changes[24,37] implying that such restrictions may affect changes that occur with aging. Age has also been found to be associated with a decline in the number of villi and crypts, loss of villi and enterocyte height, and decline in mucosal surface.[24] However, a clear association between intestinal morphology and nutrient uptake with aging has yet to be shown.[24,38]

MALNUTRITION STATES AS THEY RELATE TO AGING

Pathologic protein-energy malnutrition usually arises when there are disease states superimposed on normal aging. Certain undernutrition syndromes may be clinically apparent and consistent with the patient's presenting diagnosis. **Table 1**[1,39,40] depicts such presentations. These are distinct entities, but they are not mutually exclusive.

ASSESSING NUTRITIONAL RISK IN THE GERIATRIC SURGICAL PATIENT
History, Physical Examination, and Supporting Laboratory Results

The first step in the assessment of the patient's nutritional status is a thorough history and physical examination. Classifying a patient as being well nourished based on a cursory examination of weight or body mass index (BMI) and a serum albumin level is incomplete and often incorrect.[16] Supporting laboratory investigations are important but should be used with caution. For example, a low albumin or prealbumin level may be caused by malnutrition, but it can also be a marker of inflammation and catabolism in disease.[16] A malnourished patient may have a normal serum albumin level, or, conversely, a well-nourished patient may have a low serum albumin level. Furthermore, in high-acuity states, catabolism may simply be an adaptive response to acute illness, which may again illicit a low serum albumin level, which is clearly not reflective of their nutritional state.[16,41,42]

A history and physical examination should capture some basic information. One should evaluate the patient's history for recent unexplained weight loss. Medical history such as depression, dementia, neurologic disease, chronic infections, gastrointestinal disorders including reflux, malignancy, and neurologic, endocrine, and end-organ disease should be collected. Surgical history of gastrointestinal reconstruction (ie, intestinal resection, gastric bypass) is also important to note. Furthermore, special attention to common problems in the elderly is warranted.[43] In general, depression is the most common cause of malnutrition[43] in the elderly followed by malignancy. Routine assessment for signs and symptoms of depression

Table 1		
Case presentations and pathophysiology (in brief) of undernutrition syndromes		
Undernutrition Syndrome	**Case Presentation**	**Pathophysiology**
Anorexia	79 y-old Mrs X reports that she just does not feel like eating. Her favorite foods are no longer enticing. She reports that this began after the death of her husband a year ago. She cries as she reports this to you.	Anorexia is a decrease in appetite. Older adults are more predisposed. Depression is a frequent cause.[1] Other causes include drug side effects, dementia, and illness.[1] Anorexia may be related to gastrointestinal changes, hormonal changes, and sensory changes.[1] Differentiate from unable to eat because of dysphagia, food insecurity, denture problems, or other potentially reversible causes.
Cachexia	55 y-old Mr Y is a known patient with pancreatic cancer. He has unresectable disease and is receiving chemoradiotherapy. He reports a drop of 20 kg in 3 mo. He appears muscle wasted, emaciated, frail, and has reduced hair. He complains of fatigue, anorexia, early satiety, taste and smell disturbance, and nausea.	Cachexia is characterized by profound loss (up to 80%) of adipose tissue and skeletal muscle mass, which is associated with hematologic derangements and asthenia.[39] It is a complex syndrome characterized by inflammation and altered metabolism[39] and is associated with metabolic disease, cancer, acquired immunodeficiency syndrome, or end-stage organ disease.
Sarcopenia	75-y-old Mr Z is said to be shrinking, he has smaller muscles and feels generally weaker than 5 y prior. Otherwise, he is in good health, he has just had a routine medical checkup that came out normal.	Sarcopenia is the loss of muscle mass accompanied by decreased strength that is associated with age.[40] It is related to reductions in androgenic hormones, insulin resistance, decreased physical activity, and reduced protein intake.[40] It is accompanied by weakness and may lead to functional disability and falls if severe.[40]

Data from Refs.[1,39,40]

are extremely important.[44] In addition, a thorough physical examination of the skin, hair, oral mucosa, and tongue may provide critical information about the hydration and nutrition status of the geriatric patient.[45]

Calculation of Nutritional Risk

The American Society for Parenteral and Enteral Nutrition and the American Diabetes Association have recently recommended a standardized set of diagnostic criteria to be used to identify and document adult malnutrition. If the patient has 2 of the following, he or she has malnutrition: insufficient energy intake, recent weight loss, loss of muscle mass, loss of subcutaneous fat, localized or generalized fluid accumulation, and diminished functional status as measured by hand grip strength.[16] The hand strength test with a dynamometer has the strongest correlation with muscle mass and nutritional status among physical function assessments. It is logical to presume that in the quick assessment of a hospitalized patient with many pressing health and management issues, the above assessment may be limited because of relative physician expertise, and reproducibility may be compromised by competing factors such as hydration status.

Determining a patient's risk for malnutrition would be key during the preoperative visit to plan and optimize supportive measures accordingly.[17,46] The Malnutrition Screening Tool (MST) is a quick and easy tool to help determine this risk, as it asks 2 simple questions: "Have you been eating poorly because of a decreased appetite?" and "Have you lost weight recently without trying?," and it is accurate when compared with the standard Subjective Global Assessment.[17] The MST is reliable and sensitive and may be used to screen patients for the need for further nutritional assessment. One must elicit reasons for difficulty eating. These reasons may have medical treatments available if recognized, such as dysphagia, poorly fitting dentures, intention tremor, or rigidity.

Additional tools are also available for conducting nutritional assessments. The Short Nutritional Assessment Questionnaire is similar to the MST; it is validated and practical.[47,48] The Mini Nutritional assessment (MNA) has the advantage that it is designed for use in the elderly population.[49] It can also detect malnutrition when BMI and albumin levels are within normal ranges. The MNA has a brief screening assessment that can identify an at-risk patient, and a full or complete MNA can be completed in 10 to 15 minutes.[49] However, the presence of comorbidities may be considered in addition to the MNA result.[19] The MNA is widely cited as a screening tool and is validated in an acutely hospitalized patient.[49] It can be used for follow-up to determine the effect of an intervention.[49] The forms for these screening tools are widely available on the internet[49] and in the American Diabetes Association pocket guide to nutritional assessment.[50] It is advised that some form of nutritional screening be done and that the method used is documented for future reference and to ensure that appropriate follow-up, such as dietician consultation, is conducted.

In addition to clinically recognizable nutritional deficiency syndromes, a clinician often predicts or forms an opinion on the degree of surgical risk just by visiting the patient for the first time. The opinion is usually that the patient looks well for his age or looks fragile for his age.[3] However, this assessment may not be a sufficient valuation of surgical risk. Instead, the Portsmouth Physiological and Operative Severity Score for the Enumeration of Mortality and Morbidity (P-POSSUM) score may be calculated. It is obtained by entering 12 widely available physiologic parameters into an equation and can be modified using basic intraoperative parameters, which can be done using online calculators.[51] The result is a percentage risk of morbidity or mortality at 30 days. This score is validated for use in general surgery patients and is also available for risk-adjusted analysis.[52] There are limitations when using this score in healthy subjects, as it may be grossly overestimated even after the P-POSSUM adjustment.[52]

Calculating nutritional risk using unfiltered laboratory assessments may be misleading in elderly surgical patients. A more accurate choice would be the Geriatric Nutritional Index Score.[53] This score incorporates weight, a surrogate for height, and serum albumin level in the nutritional risk assessment of acute elderly hospitalized patients. This score has been found to be accurate in establishing the risk of complications and death associated with elderly patients' nutritional status.[53] Because the usual weight and height of the patient are not always known or easily measurable for an elderly individual because of decreased mobility or poor memory, height and usual weight are not used. Instead the calculation is based on knee height, ideal weight (as calculated by the Lorentz equation), and serum albumin level entered into a simple equation. The score thresholds correlate with a 5% and 10% weight loss and albumin thresholds of 38, 35, and 30 and predict mortality and complication-ridden survival at 6 months.[53] In addition, BMI less than 19, albumin level less than 3.0, and weight loss in excess of 5%[17] and 10%[41] are known predictors of poor survival. BMI less than 18.5 in an adult[54] and less than 20 in an older adult are independent predictors of mortality in intensive care unit patients.[55] Laboratory measurements of prealbumin, transferrin, and retinol-binding protein levels can assess for acute starvation, but no value should stand alone.[41]

An association has been described between higher BMI and surviving critical illness,[54] but this assertion requires further research.[56] There is additional evidence that overweight and mildly obese elderly individuals have longer survival rates in general.[1,57,58] As data continue to accrue, it may be found that overweight elderly individuals have better odds of surviving an intensive care unit stay. Therefore, weight loss in an elderly patient should be an individually based decision, which carefully considers expected quality of life changes in association with the patient's comorbidities.

Promoting Dietary Intake and Setting Reasonable Goals

Elderly individuals should receive special attention regarding the status of their overall process of eating and digestion. Simple factors such as poor dentition or mal-fitting dentures may impact their ability to consume a meal. Difficulty swallowing may lead to silent aspiration or fear of consuming certain foods. The frequency and severity of gastrointestinal upsets, bowel movement patterns, or constipation may impact food choices or volume.[43] A preemptive understanding of the possible challenges to maintain an appropriate diet in an acutely hospitalized individual may help caregivers ensure the appropriate intake during hospitalization. An effort should be made to know whether the patient has true food intolerances,[57] food preferences, or specific food dislikes such that the caregiver team may provide adequate and effective nutrition for the patient.

Restrictive diets in this population are cautioned against because they have been associated with increased risk of malnutrition.[57] Recommendations to suit chronic diseases should involve monitoring and continual management instead of strict exclusions[57] (ie, measure effects of sweets on glycemia and institute appropriate insulin protocol instead of cutting out all concentrated sweets). It is also important to not remove all salt from hypertensive geriatric patients' diets,[57] because of the palatability of food and the dizziness and fall risk of hypovolemic patients who may also be prescribed diuretics.

Multiple comorbidities are common in elderly individuals; thus, they are often prescribed multiple medications to treat these diseases. It is difficult to separate whether polypharmacy worsens malnutrition or whether these 2 occurrences coexist in the vulnerable population of the elderly, with or without medical morbidity, and social deprivation factors like food insecurity.[23,44] It should be noted, however, that medications have common side effects that may be easily overlooked, such as dyspepsia or gastrointestinal intolerance. Furthermore, certain commonly prescribed medications have side effects affecting nutritional status such as anorexia, early satiety, reduced ability to eat, dysphagia, constipation, and diarrhea. If an elderly patient is feeling off balance because of medication-induced dizziness, nausea, or myalgias, it is also reasonable to believe that he or she would eat less. In addition, in elderly patients who take multiple medications (often up to 10 or more), possible side effects may be difficult to identify and may be superimposed by drug interactions.[44] A thorough review of symptoms may help capture missed gastrointestinal disturbances or side effects of medications in an elderly individual.

It is important that recent weight loss is identified and quantified when possible during the preoperative visit.[16] Availability of serial weight measurements are preferred, as they may reflect a trend that may more readily identify malnutrition. Once recognized, malnutrition or weight loss should be communicated to all health care professionals involved in the patient's care. In addition, weight should be plotted against estimated weight for age and height on an available weight chart, because the number alone may be misinterpreted by clinicians, and those whose number is less than 80% of expected weight may be considered underweight. Treating physicians should be cognizant that even if a proper diet is instituted and successful, weight gain in the elderly is slower compared with their younger counterparts.

The Provision of Nutrients to Elderly Critically Ill Surgical Patients

Overview of nutrient delivery

When an elderly patient requires tube feedings or total parenteral nutrition, the clinical care provider must evaluate all factors involved with providing adequate nutrition for their patient. This evaluation entails the assessment of their basal and total energy expenditure, type of and amount of calories needed to achieve goal calories, and the delivering of other necessary vitamins and adjuncts. One must also consider the method of delivery (enteral vs parenteral) and patient-specific access (central vs peripheral total parenteral nutrition, gastric vs postpyloric or jejunal) and complications associated with each of these. Continuous assessment is needed to ensure that the individual is neither overfed nor underfed.

The provision of calories by artificial means is often necessary in critically ill surgical patients. The enteral route is preferred whenever possible, via nasogastric tube, gastrostomy, or jejunostomy, as clinically applicable. Precautions should be taken to avoid aspiration, as elderly individuals are generally at increased risk. When indicated, enteral nutrition should be started 1 to 2 days after admission. If illness is not expected to last longer than 3 to 5 days in a well-nourished individual or 5 to 7 days in a poorly nourished individual, artificial nutrition, whether enteral or parenteral, may be unnecessary. The provision of calories sufficient to meet caloric needs is calculated based on height, weight, activity, and nature of stress. The provision of nutrients is titrated clinically.

In the case that an elderly individual is suspected to have low oral intake, especially while acutely hospitalized, a search for the reason of poor intake should ensue. For individuals admitted without a gastrointestinal complaint, current dysphagia and previous insult to the cricopharyngeal mechanism are worth ruling out. Disorders that affect the cricopharyngeal mechanism of swallowing are many and include neurologic disorders such as previous stroke, Parkinsonism, esophageal motility disorders, gastroesophageal reflux, and mechanical obstruction caused by cancer or something else. Patients may present because of recurrent episodes of aspiration, which raises the suspicion for disorders affecting swallowing or cough reflex.[59] For individuals found to have decreased oral intake because of mechanical difficulties associated with a medical condition and who are determined to be malnourished or at risk of malnourishment after nutritional assessment, the placement of a percutaneous endoscopic gastrostomy must be entertained. Proper discussion should we done with the patient and the family to come to that decision, and it is preferable that it be for individuals with moderate-to-good prognosis.

Nutrient requirements

The most accurate method to calculate the basal energy expenditure is the Harris-Benedict equation, which is based on height, weight, gender, and age. For an initial estimate of total energy expenditure, one must multiply by the appropriate activity factor of the patient and by the appropriate stress factor.[60] Therefore, careful assessment must be made of the mitigating factors for nutritional requirement, such as sepsis, fever, inflammation, surgical trauma, or traumatic long bone fractures, which would factor into increased stress.

As a general rule, an individual should receive 25 kcal/kg/d in an unstressed situation. One then must multiply this amount by the activity and stress factors to estimate requirements in a hospitalized patient.[61] Protein requirements are also increased by stress and are thus important to counteract the loss of lean muscle mass in a postoperative patient. Counteracting the loss of lean muscle mass may be especially important in the elderly. There are no specific protein recommendations for artificial nutrition supplied to the elderly, but 0.8 g/kg/d is the current recommendation for adults and is increased with stress and protein losing conditions.[61] In patients with end-stage renal disease on dialysis, greater than the usual dose of protein is recommended. Patients on continuous renal replacement therapy should receive 2.5 times the usual amount of protein.[62,63] In patients with end-stage renal disease not on dialysis, the normal amount for an unstressed patient is recommended. Patients with renal disease should receive less to none of certain trace elements. Patients with liver disease should receive about the usual amount of protein.[63] A patient with liver-related encephalopathy that is refractory to medical management may benefit from branched-chain amino acids.[62,63]

Micronutrients are slowly being recognized as therapies, as they may be conditionally essential in conditions of disease, such as arginine and glutamine.[64] Furthermore, selenium, a trace element with antioxidant properties, has shown potential for a direct therapeutic effect when given in doses beyond the recommended daily values.[61,64,65] The use of micronutrients as therapy is an active avenue of research. Not enough is known about trace element status in the elderly to make recommendations for this age group.[66] Ergogenic diets have not been studied sufficiently in the elderly to make recommendations.[67] Biological mechanisms at the cellular level are being evaluated to perhaps detect the effect of micronutrients on aging and to detect the effect of nutritional interventions.[68]

Clinicians must be aware of the possibility of symptomatic micronutrient deficiency states developing in patients, especially in those individuals who are predisposed because of chronic malnutrition. However, deficiency states usually do not develop because of body stores when patients are on artificial nutrition for less than 3 months.[69] Patients with certain diseases are more likely to have deficiency in certain nutrients, such as zinc in cases of increased gastrointestinal loss,[69] but despite its reported positive effect on healing, it is not recommended in excess.[64] Although iron is deficient in critical illness and is needed for erythropoiesis, there are theoretic concerns over its safety, including the association with sepsis and an altered redox potential in the cells. In addition, iron supplementation has not been proven to prevent the need for transfusion.[70]

Type of formulation

Different formulations for enteral feeding exist. Patients with normal to near-normal digesting ability can receive polymeric feedings. Patients with malabsorption syndromes require elemental or predigested feedings. Fiber supplemented feedings are contraindicated before full resuscitation and restoration of hemodynamic stability and in patients who have dysmotility or who are predisposed to bowel ischemia.[62] Soluble fiber may be indicated in patients without a contraindication who have diarrhea.[62,64] A combination of antioxidant vitamins and trace minerals is recommended in both enteral and parenteral regimens. The exact composition of micronutrients is under debate because of manufacturing limitations and the absence of recommendations for dosage, specifically determined for elderly critically ill surgical patients.

Immune-modulating enteral formulations have been shown to be beneficial in surgical critically ill patients.[11,62] These formulations contain arginine, glutamine, nucleic acids, omega 3 fatty acids, and vitamin antioxidants. There is some evidence that immune-modulating formulations should not be given to patients who are already severely septic.[62] There is also evidence for enteral glutamine alone in burn, trauma, and mixed critically ill patients.[62] Patients with acute respiratory distress syndrome should be placed on anti-inflammatory lipid formulations.[62] There is some evidence for the use of probiotics in patients with major abdominal surgeries, transplants, and severe trauma, but no general recommendation can be made.[62] Intravenous lipid emulsions seem to help in sepsis and in preventing end-organ failure in this setting, whereas enteral fish oils are still under study.[61] No specific high-level recommendations are made regarding indications and recommended doses for individual micronutrients in artificial nutrition for critical care patients and for the elderly subgroup.

Glycemic control

The institution of feeding in a critically ill patient may have a negative effect on glycemic control. The maintenance of normoglycemia must be maintained in all patients, including those receiving artificial nutrition.[62] Special attention must be given to times of stoppage of feeding for procedures and changes in rate of feeding to prevent variations in glycemia and episodes of hypoglycemia. Overfeeding should be avoided. Hyperglycemia in critically ill patients is associated with an increased risk of infections, length of stay, dependence on organ support, and overall mortality.[71] Hyperglycemia is detrimental to immune functions and promotes infection[72]; furthermore, it is theorized that maintenance of normoglycemia may help reverse the systemic inflammatory immune response. The amalgamation of the largest clinical trial proposes that strictest control of hyperglycemia without causing episodes of hypoglycemia is associated with the best outcome.[73] Although the initial value and trend of glycemia may of prognostic value,[74] there is sufficient evidence to believe that achieving and maintaining normoglycemia is of significant benefit to outcome in a critically ill elderly hospitalized patient.[75] The authors suggest that a sliding scale of intravenous insulin be instituted, perhaps similar to the modified Yale protocol, with special guidance at the time of instituting and stopping feedings and validated at every institution for safety.

For diabetic elderly individuals, the same percentage of carbohydrates in artificial nutrition may be used or slightly less at 30% to 40% of the total caloric requirements, instead of the usual 50% of total requirements. Use of oral antihyperglycemic drugs is discouraged because of the risk of hypoglycemia. Metformin use is discouraged because it increases the risk of lactic acidosis in septic patients and in those who receive intravenous contrast. Control of glycemia in diabetics on parenteral nutrition may require more than their usual amount of insulin.[41]

Common vitamin deficiencies

Because of impaired processes necessary for production of vitamin D in aging adults and because deficiency is associated with depression, cognitive impairment, and increased risk of fractures, adequate vitamin D intake is recommended. The recommended dietary allowance (RDA) of vitamin D for adults through age 70 years is 600 IU with the recommended dietary allowance increasing to 800 IU after age 71. Patients who are institutionalized are at particular risk for vitamin D deficiency because of poor exposure to sunlight. Vitamin D is not sufficiently studied for use in intensive care,[76] although acute cases of symptomatic bone loss caused by vitamin D deficiency associated with parenteral nutrition are reported.[69]

Patients at risk for vitamin B12 deficiency because of previous gastric surgery or gastric disease or those who have neurologic, psychological, and hematologic disturbances determined to be caused by vitamin B12 should be supplemented with oral B12 at a 1000 μg/d. Because of extensive physiologic stores, vitamin B12 deficiency will not set in clinically for a few years after absorption ceases, so replacement only becomes important in long-term states of deficiency such as surgical gastrectomies or pernicious anemia, or when a deficiency state is otherwise diagnosed if suspected.

If it is deemed that an elderly individual may be unable to achieve micronutrient recommended requirements because of poor intake, it may be prudent to prescribe a multivitamin. However, the National Institutes of Health Census in 2006 did not find sufficient evidence to recommend for or against routine prescription of a multivitamin to elderly individuals.

GENERAL IN-HOSPITAL RECOMMENDATIONS FOR NUTRITION OF ELDERLY SURGICAL PATIENTS
General Recommendations

- Every patient should receive at least a brief nutritional assessment[41] at admission[16] in accordance with hospital policy and useful to allied health staff. The assessment performed should be documented in the medical chart and the nutritional status continually communicated to treating physicians as more information is available.[41] If the patient is malnourished or at risk of malnourishment according to the initial screening tools (MST, the Short Nutritional Assessment Questionnaire, MNA) or according to the assessment of his or her physician, formal dietary assessment should be initiated.
- When an elderly surgical patient is prescribed a diet, every effort should be made by the caring physician, nurse, and allied health professionals to ensure that the diet prescribed is provided to and successfully received by the patient. Any issues with access[21] and palatability should be reported to the caring team, and a search for alternatives should occur. This search requires attention to possible physical limitations of the elderly individual.[41]
- Hospitalized patients should be assessed regularly for medical signs of nutritional intolerance such nausea, vomiting, pain, difficulty chewing or swallowing, impaired bowel function, and physical signs of intolerance on physical and abdominal examination.

Continued Assessment

- After the initial nutritional assessment, if the patient is at increased risk for malnutrition, further specialized testing will occur by consulted allied health care professionals. The information and recommendations ensuing should be discussed with the team, including the attending physician.[16]
- Any nutritional intervention should be monitored for efficacy and modified as needed.

- The patient's bowel movements should be managed consistently.[77] For instance, if the patient takes a laxative at home, this should not be withdrawn for longer than necessary after surgery, and one should not wait for the development of constipation. If a patient is given a medication that can cause constipation, the appropriate kind and strength of prophylactic laxative should be added and tailored to the individual patient's bowel pattern and response to medication. If a patient gets diarrhea, other than the usual medical intervention and workup, efforts should be made to modify the diet to decrease the problem without withdrawing nutrition, when possible. If the patient is expected to have nausea because of his medical or surgical treatment, protocols immediately available at the bedside should address the symptoms targeting immediate relief and then triggering a formal evaluation.

Enteral Nutrition

- Tolerance to the method of nutrition must be assessed.[77] Decisions for nutrition are important medical decisions that are often life changing and should be discussed with the elderly person involved and his family when appropriate. An elderly person may have increased issues with tolerance to the nutritional method of access chosen and many opt out of it altogether. It is important to define goals of care.[62]
- The type of nutrition provided should be chosen mindfully. No specific recommendation exists for the elderly, but the closest to physiologic may be wise unless contraindicated, for example, fiber-rich enteral nutrition.[77] The proportion of calories to be supplied as carbohydrates, proteins, and fat in parenteral nutrition should be standard and may be approached regularly to respond to the patient's clinical course by the nutritionist and the clinical team.
- The provision of micronutrients must be considered for every patient, including the amount necessary, whether certain micronutrients may be beneficial in excess amounts, and the avoidance of toxic levels by adjusting for comorbid conditions. If nutrition is enteral, it is suggested that the whole requirement for micronutrient is provided even if less-than-usual calories are provided.
- Monitoring of electrolyte imbalances is done as appropriate to the clinical condition of the patient[77] and more aggressively if the patient is at risk for refeeding syndrome.
- Fluid balance is important in an elderly individual.[77] Large shifts in fluid status are discouraged. Special attention should be given for underlying pathologies, such as heart failure. The elderly's kidney concentrating capacity is less than that of a young adult, so adequate amounts of water should be considered. The amount of fluid given with nutrition may be limited by the necessary medical restriction of fluids in certain elderly individuals.
- The risk of aspiration is larger in elderly individuals,[77] so precautions must be assiduously followed.
- The interference with drug absorption is possible, and previous control may be altered by the new provision of nutrition. Monitoring should occur as clinically indicated; for example, monitoring of anticoagulant levels should be considered.
- The clinician must be aware of the possibility of malabsorption syndromes. The specific history and clinical course will guide appropriate workup and intervention.
- Glycemic goals must be defined,[77] and changes appropriate in magnitude to the clinical situation should be instituted to shift smoothly toward euglycemia.

- Elderly should be assessed regularly for the ability to return to an oral diet.[77] Perceived readiness should prompt a monitored trial of oral diet.

Parenteral Nutrition

- The clinician must be mindful of complications of vascular access (ie, central line sepsis) and monitor accordingly. Regular follow-up should be done to ensure the supply of an adequate amount of nutrients without metabolic consequences (ie, liver failure).
- Elderly individuals may exhibit early sepsis differently than younger adults.
- Fluid, electrolyte, and micronutrient supplementation should be tailored clinically the individual.
- Glycemic goals must be defined, and changes appropriate in magnitude to the clinical situation should be instituted to shift smoothly toward euglycemia.
- Elderly should be regularly assessed for the ability to return to an oral diet. Perceived readiness should prompt a monitored trial of oral diet.

The Relationship of Drugs and Nutrition

- The hospitalization period may serve to optimize the patient's medications, to observe for wanted effects, and to control for unwanted ones. Consultation should be considered when a medication is suspected to cause harm but treats an active clinical condition.
- Consider STOPP (Screening Tool of Older Persons' potentially inappropriate Prescriptions) and START (Screening Tool to Alert doctors to Right Treatment) criteria for medications that seem to be producing significant side-effects that can impact nutritional status. For example, opioids can be replaced with acetaminophen if the pain is not severe.
- Especially when new medications are started, it is advisable to monitor for side effects that can affect dietary intake.

Discharge Planning

- On discharge planning, it is wise to flag a patient who is nutritionally at risk or who has received in-house nutritional interventions, such that nutritional assessment for undernutrition may not be missed on follow-up visits.[16,41] A patient may have food insecurity that is unmasked because of new dietary restrictions that are prescribed or related to the consequences of surgical disease or chronic hospitalization. A worsened nutritional status may lead to a spiral of clinical deterioration.
- For individuals who may be discharged on enteral and parenteral nutrition, early arrangements should be made for professional home care and adequate follow-up.

In general, it is important that the clinical care team identify problems that can be quickly remedied to ensure adequate nutritional intake. It would also be wise to emulate the patient's nutritional habits from home if those were working for the patient, such as home cooking to be brought in by family. In addition, ensuring a comfortable environment for eating and the exact amount of help necessary to allow the patient autonomy of eating when possible would help to improve the patient's intake. For every kind of nutrition provided, whether oral, enteral, or parenteral, special care must be taken to monitor for the complications common in the elderly population.

SUMMARY

Elderly people experience physiologic changes in the gut and in every organ system, which predisposes them to impaired nutrition and associated increased risk factors.

When the normal processes of aging is compounded by illness, the propensity to cause a pathologic state of malnutrition increases. Surgical nutrition support in the critical care setting aims to identify those at nutritional risk and to support nutritional needs in the direction of recovery. New evidence has arisen for use of certain nutrients as therapeutic agents because they are thought to contribute to the healing process and may be conditionally deficient in stress related to disease processes. Nutritional support is critical to the successful surgical outcome in the geriatric surgical population. It is important that health care providers follow evidenced-based recommendations for the provision of adequate nutrients and address the individual needs of every patient.

REFERENCES

1. Morley JE. Pathophysiology of the anorexia of aging. Curr Opin Clin Nutr Metab Care 2013;16(1):27–32.
2. Chapman IM. The anorexia of aging. Clin Geriatr Med 2007;23(4):735–56, v.
3. Farquharson SM, Gupta R, Heald RJ, et al. Surgical decisions in the elderly: the importance of biological age. J R Soc Med 2001;94(5):232–5.
4. Dudrick SJ. Nutrition management of geriatric surgical patients. Surg Clin North Am 2011;91(4):877–96, ix.
5. Oresanya LB, Lyons WL, Finlayson E. Preoperative assessment of the older patient: a narrative review. JAMA 2014;311(20):2110–20.
6. Makary MA, Segev DL, Pronovost PJ, et al. Frailty as a predictor of surgical outcomes in older patients. J Am Coll Surg 2010;210(6):901–8.
7. Robinson TN, Wallace JI, Wu DS, et al. Accumulated frailty characteristics predict postoperative discharge institutionalization in the geriatric patient. J Am Coll Surg 2011;213(1):37–42 [discussion: 42–4].
8. Kristjansson SR, Farinella E, Gaskell S, et al. Surgical risk and post-operative complications in older unfit cancer patients. Cancer Treat Rev 2009;35(6):499–502.
9. Ortman JM. Presentation for the FFC/GW. BrownBag Seminar Series on Forecasting, February 7, 2013. Washington (DC): United States Census Bureau.
10. Sealey G. U.S elderly to double in 25 years, in A.B.C news. ABC News internet ventures; 2014.
11. Culebras JM. Malnutrition in the twenty-first century: an epidemic affecting surgical outcome. Surg Infect (Larchmt) 2013;14(3):237–43.
12. Yang R, Wolfson M, Lewis MC. Unique aspects of the elderly surgical population: an anesthesiologist's perspective. Geriatr Orthop Surg Rehabil 2011;2(2):56–64.
13. Number of all-listed procedures for discharges from short-stay hospitals, by procedure category and age, N.H.D. Survey, editor. 2010: United States.
14. Kwag SJ, Kim JG, Kang WK, et al. The nutritional risk is a independent factor for postoperative morbidity in surgery for colorectal cancer. Ann Surg Treat Res 2014;86(4):206–11.
15. Nozoe T, Kimura Y, Ishida M, et al. Correlation of pre-operative nutritional condition with post-operative complications in surgical treatment for oesophageal carcinoma. Eur J Surg Oncol 2002;28(4):396–400.
16. White JV, Guenter P, Jensen G, et al. Consensus statement of the Academy of Nutrition and Dietetics/American Society for Parenteral and Enteral Nutrition: characteristics recommended for the identification and documentation of adult malnutrition (undernutrition). J Acad Nutr Diet 2012;112(5):730–8.
17. Almeida AI, Correia M, Camilo M, et al. Nutritional risk screening in surgery: valid, feasible, easy! Clin Nutr 2012;31(2):206–11.

18. Morgan TM, Tang D, Stratton KL, et al. Preoperative nutritional status is an important predictor of survival in patients undergoing surgery for renal cell carcinoma. Eur Urol 2011;59(6):923–8.
19. Vischer UM, Frangos E, Graf C, et al. The prognostic significance of malnutrition as assessed by the Mini Nutritional Assessment (MNA) in older hospitalized patients with a heavy disease burden. Clin Nutr 2012;31(1):113–7.
20. Schricker T, Wykes L, Meterissian S, et al. The anabolic effect of perioperative nutrition depends on the patient's catabolic state before surgery. Ann Surg 2013;257(1):155–9.
21. Bell AF, Walton K, Chevis JS, et al. Accessing packaged food and beverages in hospital. Exploring experiences of patients and staff. Appetite 2013;60(1): 231–8.
22. Ji L, Meng H, Dong B. Factors associated with poor nutritional status among the oldest-old. Clin Nutr 2012;31(6):922–6.
23. Sattler EL, Lee JS. Persistent food insecurity is associated with higher levels of cost-related medication nonadherence in low-income older adults. J Nutr Gerontol Geriatr 2013;32(1):41–58.
24. Ahmed T, Haboubi N. Assessment and management of nutrition in older people and its importance to health. Clin Interv Aging 2010;5:207–16.
25. Saffrey MJ. Ageing of the enteric nervous system. Mech Ageing Dev 2004; 125(12):899–906.
26. Cowen T, Johnson RJ, Soubeyre V, et al. Restricted diet rescues rat enteric motor neurones from age related cell death. Gut 2000;47(5):653–60.
27. Santer RM, Baker DM. Enteric neuron numbers and sizes in Auerbach's plexus in the small and large intestine of adult and aged rats. J Auton Nerv Syst 1988; 25(1):59–67.
28. Fich A, Camilleri M, Phillips SF. Effect of age on human gastric and small bowel motility. J Clin Gastroenterol 1989;11(4):416–20.
29. Bitar KN, Patil SB. Aging and gastrointestinal smooth muscle. Mech Ageing Dev 2004;125(12):907–10.
30. Elphick HL, Elphick DA, Sanders DS. Small bowel bacterial overgrowth. An under-recognized cause of malnutrition in older adults. Geriatrics 2006;61(9):21–6.
31. Parlesak A, Klein B, Schecher K, et al. Prevalence of small bowel bacterial overgrowth and its association with nutrition intake in nonhospitalized older adults. J Am Geriatr Soc 2003;51(6):768–73.
32. Gullo L, Ventrucci M, Naldoni P, et al. Aging and exocrine pancreatic function. J Am Geriatr Soc 1986;34(11):790–2.
33. Laugier R, Bernard JP, Berthezene P, et al. Changes in pancreatic exocrine secretion with age: pancreatic exocrine secretion does decrease in the elderly. Digestion 1991;50(3–4):202–11.
34. Dreiling DA, Triebling AT, Koller M. The effect of age on human exocrine pancreatic secretion. Mt Sinai J Med 1985;52(5):336–9.
35. Popper H. Aging and the liver. Prog Liver Dis 1986;8:659–83.
36. Cao SX, Dhahbi JM, Mote PL, et al. Genomic profiling of short- and long-term caloric restriction effects in the liver of aging mice. Proc Natl Acad Sci U S A 2001;98(19):10630–5.
37. Drozdowski L, Thomson AB. Aging and the intestine. World J Gastroenterol 2006; 12(47):7578–84.
38. Keelan M, Walker K, Thomson AB. Intestinal morphology, marker enzymes and lipid content of brush border membranes from rabbit jejunum and ileum: effect of aging. Mech Ageing Dev 1985;31(1):49–68.

39. Ronga I, Gallucci F, Riccardi F, et al. Anorexia-cachexia syndrome in pancreatic cancer: recent advances and new pharmacological approach. Adv Med Sci 2014;59(1):1–6.
40. Waters DL, Baumgartner RN, Garry PJ, et al. Advantages of dietary, exercise-related, and therapeutic interventions to prevent and treat sarcopenia in adult patients: an update. Clin Interv Aging 2010;5:259–70.
41. Guidelines for the use of parenteral and enteral nutrition in adult and pediatric patients. JPEN J Parenter Enteral Nutr 2002;26(Suppl 1):1SA–138SA.
42. Jensen GL, Bistrian B, Roubenoff R, et al. Malnutrition syndromes: a conundrum vs continuum. JPEN J Parenter Enteral Nutr 2009;33(6):710–6.
43. Cederholm T, Morley J. Ageing: biology and nutrition. Curr Opin Clin Nutr Metab Care 2013;16(1):1–2.
44. Zadak Z, Hyspler R, Ticha A, et al. Polypharmacy and malnutrition. Curr Opin Clin Nutr Metab Care 2013;16(1):50–5.
45. Ersan T. Perioperative management of the geriatric patient. Medscape; 2013 [July 28, 2014]. Available at: http://emedicine.medscape.com/article/285433-overview.
46. Lomivorotov VV, Efremov SM, Boboshko VA, et al. Prognostic value of nutritional screening tools for patients scheduled for cardiac surgery. Interact Cardiovasc Thorac Surg 2013;16(5):612–8.
47. Kruizenga HM, Seidell JC, de Vet HC, et al. Development and validation of a hospital screening tool for malnutrition: the short nutritional assessment questionnaire (SNAQ). Clin Nutr 2005;24(1):75–82.
48. Mueller C, Compher C, Ellen DM. A.S.P.E.N. clinical guidelines: nutrition screening, assessment, and intervention in adults. JPEN J Parenter Enteral Nutr 2011;35(1):16–24.
49. Guigoz Y. The Mini Nutritional Assessment (MNA) review of the literature–what does it tell us? J Nutr Health Aging 2006;10(6):466–85 [discussion: 485–7].
50. Charney P, Malone A. ADA pocket guide to nutrition assessment. 2nd edition. Chicago (IL): American Dietetic Association; 2004.
51. Smith JJ. P.P.T. Risk prediction in surgery: P-POSSUM scoring. [2001-2003 July 26, 2014 July 26, 2014]. Available at: http://www.riskprediction.org.uk/pp-index.php. Accessed July 26, 2014.
52. Mohil RS, Bhatnagar D, Bahadur L, et al. POSSUM and P-POSSUM for risk-adjusted audit of patients undergoing emergency laparotomy. Br J Surg 2004; 91(4):500–3.
53. Bouillanne O, Morineau G, Dupont C, et al. Geriatric Nutritional Risk Index: a new index for evaluating at-risk elderly medical patients. Am J Clin Nutr 2005;82(4): 777–83.
54. Pickkers P, de Keizer N, Dusseljee J, et al. Body mass index is associated with hospital mortality in critically ill patients: an observational cohort study. Crit Care Med 2013;41(8):1878–83.
55. Garrouste-Orgeas M, Troché G, Azoulay E, et al. Body mass index. An additional prognostic factor in ICU patients. Intensive Care Med 2004;30(3):437–43.
56. Kiraly L, Hurt RT, Van Way CW 3rd. The outcomes of obese patients in critical care. JPEN J Parenter Enteral Nutr 2011;35(Suppl 5):29S–35S.
57. Zeanandin G, Molato O, Le Duff F, et al. Impact of restrictive diets on the risk of undernutrition in a free-living elderly population. Clin Nutr 2012;31(1): 69–73.
58. Stessman J, Jacobs JM, Ein-Mor E, et al. Normal body mass index rather than obesity predicts greater mortality in elderly people: the Jerusalem longitudinal study. J Am Geriatr Soc 2009;57(12):2232–8.

59. Clave P, Rofes L, Carrión S, et al. Pathophysiology, relevance and natural history of oropharyngeal dysphagia among older people. Nestle Nutr Inst Workshop Ser 2012;72:57–66.
60. Jacobs DG, Jacobs DO, Kudsk KA, et al. Practice management guidelines for nutritional support of the trauma patient. J Trauma 2004;57(3):660–78 [discussion: 679].
61. Chambrier C, Barnoud D. How to feed complicated patients after surgery: what's new? Curr Opin Crit Care 2014;20(4):438–43.
62. McClave SA, Martindale RG, Vanek VW, et al. Guidelines for the provision and assessment of nutrition support therapy in the adult critically ill patient: Society of Critical Care Medicine (SCCM) and American Society for Parenteral and Enteral Nutrition (A.S.P.E.N.). JPEN J Parenter Enteral Nutr 2009;33(3):277–316.
63. Martindale RG, McClave SA, Vanek VW, et al. Guidelines for the provision and assessment of nutrition support therapy in the adult critically ill patient: Society of Critical Care Medicine and American Society for parenteral and enteral nutrition: executive summary. Crit Care Med 2009;37(5):1757–61.
64. Hayes GL, McKinzie BP, Bullington WM, et al. Nutritional supplements in critical illness. AACN Adv Crit Care 2011;22(4):301–16 [quiz: 317–8].
65. Heyland DK. Selenium supplementation in critically ill patients: can too much of a good thing be a bad thing? Crit Care 2007;11(4):153.
66. Sfar S, El Heni J, Laporte F, et al. Trace element status and fatty acids metabolism during healthy ageing: an example of a population from the Tunisian eastern coast. Exp Gerontol 2012;47(3):243–9.
67. Cherniack EP. Ergogenic dietary aids for the elderly. Nutrition 2012;28(3):225–9.
68. Soares H, Marinho HS, Real C, et al. Cellular polarity in aging: role of redox regulation and nutrition. Genes Nutr 2014;9(1):371.
69. Atkinson M, Worthley LI. Nutrition in the critically ill patient: part II. Parenteral nutrition. Crit Care Resusc 2003;5(2):121–36.
70. Lapointe M. Iron supplementation in the intensive care unit: when, how much, and by what route? Crit Care 2004;8(Suppl 2):S37–41.
71. van den Berghe G, Wouters P, Weekers F, et al. Intensive insulin therapy in critically ill patients. N Engl J Med 2001;345(19):1359–67.
72. Scalea TM, Bochicchio GV, Bochicchio KM, et al. Tight glycemic control in critically injured trauma patients. Ann Surg 2007;246(4):605–10 [discussion: 610–2].
73. Finfer S, Chittock DR, Su SY, et al. Intensive versus conventional glucose control in critically ill patients. N Engl J Med 2009;360(13):1283–97.
74. Sung J, Bochicchio GV, Joshi M, et al. Admission hyperglycemia is predictive of outcome in critically ill trauma patients. J Trauma 2005;59(1):80–3.
75. Bochicchio GV, Sung J, Joshi M, et al. Persistent hyperglycemia is predictive of outcome in critically ill trauma patients. J Trauma 2005;58(5):921–4.
76. Amrein K, Venkatesh B. Vitamin D and the critically ill patient. Curr Opin Clin Nutr Metab Care 2012;15(2):188–93.
77. de la Torre AM, de Mateo Silleras B, Perez-Garcia A. Guidelines for nutrition support in the elderly. Public Health Nutr 2001;4(6A):1379–84.

Management of the Skin and Soft Tissue in the Geriatric Surgical Patient

David G. Greenhalgh, MD

KEYWORDS

- Skin • Burns • Geriatric • Wound healing • Chronic wounds

KEY POINTS

- Aging leads to intrinsic skin changes resulting in thinning, loss of dermal appendages, and increased fragility that increase the risk of injury and impair wound healing; the aging process can be accelerated by extrinsic factors such as exposure to sunlight.
- Disease processes that are more prevalent in the elderly, such as malnutrition, diabetes mellitus, treatments for malignancy, and vascular disease, all impair tissue repair.
- There are functional changes in aging that predispose the elderly to increased risk and an impaired ability to handle major wounds.
- Chronic wounds such as pressure ulcers and venous stasis ulcers are extremely difficult to treat.
- There are many ways to prevent chronic wounds in the elderly.

INTRODUCTION

The demographics of the United States population is shifting so that people are living longer while the birth rate has decreased. It has been predicted that by the year 2050 nearly one-third of the population will be older than 55 years.[1] Medical care will shift to treating this geriatric population so that all caregivers will need to know how to manage problems of the elderly. As people live longer the effects of aging on the tissues persist, so one must know what kinds of medical challenges will dominate care. The effects of aging on the skin are well known. The elderly not only suffer from skin changes; other illnesses such as diabetes mellitus and vascular disease affect normal wound healing. The effects of drugs that treat malignancies and other chronic illness also have profound effects on healing. Chronic wounds, such as pressure ulcers and venous stasis wounds, are more common in the elderly. One must know about these "never event" wounds to help prevent and treat them. This review describes the

Department of Surgery, Shriners Hospitals for Children Northern California, University of California, Davis Medical Center, 2425 Stockton Boulevard, Sacramento, CA 95817, USA
E-mail address: david.greenhalgh@ucmdc.ucdavis.edu

Surg Clin N Am 95 (2015) 103–114
http://dx.doi.org/10.1016/j.suc.2014.09.008
0039-6109/15/$ – see front matter © 2015 Elsevier Inc. All rights reserved.
surgical.theclinics.com

effects of aging and the environment on the structure of skin. The effects of common medical problems, malnutrition, diabetes mellitus, vascular disease, burns, and common treatments for wounds are discussed. A description of common chronic wounds is presented to assist in developing strategies for prevention and treatment.

SKIN CHANGES IN THE ELDERLY

Aging has profound effects on the skin.[2–7] The rate of change with aging is affected by both intrinsic and extrinsic factors. Intrinsic factors are those changes that occur in all people as they age, being essentially those factors that exist "within our bodies" in everyone who ages. Extrinsic factors are the "outside" changes resulting from exposure to the elements in the harsh environment. The most significant agent of change to the skin is exposure to ultraviolet light. The extrinsic factors accelerate the degenerative changes that occur naturally. It is clear that protection from the sun will slow down the classic aging changes of the skin.

Aging affects all components of the skin. The epithelium tends to thin out with aging, but this is contrasted with thickening of the epidermis with stress or sun exposure. The junction between the epidermis and dermis flattens. The reduction of size of the normal hills and valleys of the rete pegs leads to an increased risk for shearing injuries (blisters) of the epidermis. There is a reduction in the number of skin adnexa: hair follicles, oil glands, sebaceous glands, and other adnexa. With fewer glands for lubrication, the skin becomes drier and more prone to cracking. Lower lipid content in the stratum corneum reduces the barrier function of the epidermis. It is common knowledge that there is a reduction in hair follicle numbers, especially in the scalp, with aging. There are also fewer hair follicles throughout other parts of the skin.[6] Because the rate of re-epithelialization of partial-thickness wounds depends on the density of hair follicles, a reduction in their numbers slows the ability to resurface a wound. The skin re-epithelializes from both the epithelial edge of the wound and the skin adnexa.[8] The cells in the basal cell layer of the epithelium at the site of injury migrate across the viable wound edge. These basal epithelial cells are only capable of covering 1 to 2 cm from the wound edge, so the rest of the healing in a full-thickness wound is from contraction and scar formation. If the wound has hair follicles or other skin adnexa (partial-thickness), the keratinocytes migrate from the remaining adnexa (hair follicles) to resurface the wound. The greater the density of the hair follicles, the more rapid is the rate of healing. For instance, a superficial wound in the scalp will heal within 4 to 5 days as opposed to 2 to 3 weeks on the lower leg. As one ages, the hair follicles tend to degenerate so that a superficial wound in hairless skin is incapable of re-epithelialization. Caregivers will say that they "converted" to a full-thickness wound but in essence, the wound did not have the dermal adnexa needed to re-epithelialize.

The dermis is the main target of ultraviolet light damage.[2] There is loss of the normal cells populating the dermis, namely fibroblasts and immune cells, which impair the skin's immune function. The dermis also becomes thinner and has significant alterations in the structure of its collagen. The collagen becomes larger, more fragmented, and more disorganized. Elastin persists but becomes more fragmented. Skin loses its tensile strength and is more prone to tearing.[9] It is well known that skin becomes looser, more wrinkled, and sags with the passage of time. One advantage of looser skin, however, is that the elderly can "contract" a full-thickness wound with less interference of function (contracture).

There are many other changes in the skin with aging. There tends to be a loss of sensation that occurs in a distal to proximal fashion, especially with cold/warm sensations.[10] Thus, the elderly are less capable of sensing an injury when it occurs. The skin loses hydration and vascularity. There is a decreased capability for angiogenesis,[2–7] which leads to delayed revascularization, and the new vessels tend to have a greater tendency to leak. This problem, in addition to impaired lymphatic drainage, predisposes skin to increased edema, a factor that further impairs healing. Skin pigmentation also changes in the elderly, with spotty areas of hyperpigmentation. There are increased mutations in the skin cells that lead to "age spots" (keratoses and nevi) with increased tendencies for developing skin cancers. In addition, persons taking antiplatelet drugs or other forms of anticoagulation have increased bruising, which leads to pigment changes arising from retained heme pigments.

Finally, there are changes beneath the dermis that influence the health of the skin. There is a tendency to lose muscle mass and subcutaneous adipose tissue that increases the risk for ischemia of the skin at bony prominences. Incontinence of urine or stool are associated with skin maceration, and accentuate the risk of skin breakdown. Reflex times are delayed in the elderly, especially when responding to a dangerous situation. Slower reflexes predispose them to injuries. It is not uncommon for the geriatric patient to state, "I have done this all my life but this time I was unable to respond quickly enough to prevent the injury." Slower response times also lead to larger and more extensive injuries, especially burns. As individuals become less capable of taking care of themselves, they are at increased risk for abuse. In sum, it is clear that time has profound effects on the skin and its ability to heal.

DISEASES IN THE ELDERLY THAT AFFECT WOUND HEALING

While aging changes the skin, wound healing is relatively unaffected even at the extremes of ages. Most people heal well unless there is some underlying disease or process that impairs healing. The factors that impair healing tend to be more common in the elderly, so the clinician needs to know which factors impair tissue repair. By understanding which factors impair healing, the surgeon can better predict which patient is at a higher risk for complications. Failure to heal not only affects the incision, but any leak from an anastomosis can lead to infection, sepsis, and, ultimately, death from multiple organ dysfunction syndrome.

Malnutrition

It has been known for nearly 100 years that malnutrition impairs healing.[11–14] Total protein/calorie malnutrition (marasmus) and protein malnutrition (kwashiorkor) both can reduce tensile strengths in incisions and reduce collagen synthesis. It is also important to note that simply initiating starvation at the time of incision will lead to altered tissue repair.[15] To make this point clinically relevant, if one performs surgery and keeps the patient from eating for a week, he or she will have decreased collagen formation and an increased risk for healing failure. If this problem is manifested by a bowel leak, there is an increased risk for abscess formation and sepsis. Because the elderly are less tolerant of complications, one must optimize their nutritional status before surgery. Aggressive perioperative nutritional support may make the difference between survival and death.

There are several vitamins and micronutrients required for optimal tissue repair. Vitamin C is required for the hydroxylation of proline or lysine in the creation of procollagen triple helices. Without the formation of these hydrogen bonds, the triple helix never forms and collagen is not synthesized.[16] Fortunately the result, scurvy, is extremely rare today. The proinflammatory vitamin A is also required for optimal healing. Supplements of vitamin A have been shown to reverse healing impairments caused by steroid use[17] and radiation.[18] Several micronutrients are essential for optimizing tissue repair. Zinc[19,20] and copper[20,21] are 2 of the best-studied minerals that affect healing. Deficiencies in either micronutrient are associated with impaired wound healing in people of all ages. There are anecdotal reports that healing can be improved with specific amino acids, but the only consistent finding from studies suggest that only arginine has the potential to augment the healing process.[22]

Diabetes Mellitus

The one disease that has the most impact on tissue repair is diabetes mellitus.[23–25] Though not strictly a disease of the elderly, it increases in prevalence with increasing age. Sobering statistics emphasize the impact that diabetes has on the healing process. Twenty percent of admissions for diabetic patients are for wound-healing problems. In their lifetimes, 25% of people suffering from diabetes will develop a foot ulcer. Fifty percent of nontraumatic amputations are related to diabetes mellitus. The classic scenario is that a diabetic patient with an insensate foot develops an unnoticed ulcer that becomes infected. Once this infection is detected, there is widespread infection that frequently requires an amputation. Even if a wound is detected early, getting that wound to heal is very difficult. Margolis and colleagues[26] collected data on the healing rate in diabetic wounds treated as controls with standard treatment in prospective, randomized trials. Only 31% of the control patients healed their ulcers within 20 weeks, and it is likely that most of the patients never healed their wounds.

There are several reasons to explain why tissue repair is impaired in persons with diabetes mellitus.[23–25] The first reason is that the incidence of peripheral vascular disease is increased in the diabetic patient. These patients suffer from both macrovascular and microvascular disease. Atherosclerosis leads to impaired oxygen delivery in the distal tissues. In addition, there is a thickening of the basement membranes of capillaries that impedes delivery of oxygen and nutrients to the tissues. The thickened basement membrane also interferes with the normal flow of water and increases edema, another factor that impairs tissue repair. If a diabetic patient develops uremia, another insult arises that impairs the healing process.[27]

The second profound factor that contributes to defective healing is the peripheral neuropathy that is commonly found in diabetes mellitus. Diabetic neuropathy progresses from distal to proximal so that the foot is typically the first site to be affected. The loss of protective sensation leads to the inability to respond to minor threats of injury. Because there is no pain, there is a tendency to allow minor wounds to become more severe. Minor changes in shoes can lead to blisters that progress to full-thickness injuries. Barsun and colleagues[28] recently published their 10-year experience with burns to the feet in 68 diabetic patients. Some developed burns while walking outside on the hot pavement, others while trying to "warm" their feet in hot water or near heaters. These patients all developed full-thickness burns that led to prolonged hospitalizations and difficulties with graft take, and several amputations were required. The effects of neuropathy on the foot are a little more complicated than expected. There is a loss of the feedback that maintains the normal arch of the foot so that there is an increase in pressure on the first or second metatarsal heads. The classic "diabetic foot ulcer" occurs on the plantar aspect of the foot at this site. There is also loss of normal sympathetic nerve function that maintains normal sweating so that the foot becomes dry and tends to crack, which leads to sites of infection.

Furthermore, there is impairment in the ability of leukocytes to respond to infections in diabetes mellitus. The thickened capillary basement membrane impairs the migratory ability of leukocytes to get to the site of an infection. Hyperglycemia also impairs their bactericidal ability. Therefore, a minor infection often spreads along the fascial planes of the foot and ultimately up the leg.

Several metabolic changes that influence immune function result from the effects of diabetes mellitus.[25,29] One of the most interesting concepts is that hyperglycemia leads to increases in glucose by-products called advanced glycosylation end-products (AGES). There is a receptor for AGES (RAGES), which detects these end-products and leads to a chronic inflammatory state. One theory is that persistent activation of the RAGES pathway leads to the chronic inflammatory state known as the metabolic syndrome.[30]

Because the impairment in tissue repair is so profound in diabetes mellitus, prevention efforts are of the utmost importance.[31,32] Clinicians should make their diabetic patients aware of the risks for wound problems in their feet. Patients should check their feet daily for problems and should be careful when wearing new shoes. There should be extra caution in diabetic patients with insensate feet. These patients should never try to warm their feet and should never walk around with bare feet. Once a wound develops, it should be aggressively treated by removing any pressure on the metatarsal heads by providing footwear that "offloads" the pressure point.[33] Studies suggest that providing exogenous growth factors or applying skin substitutes that supply growth factors may improve the ability to heal, but such an approach is highly expensive.[34–36]

Therapies that Alter Wound Healing

Optimal healing requires the rapid migration of inflammatory cells to the site of injury, rapid cellular proliferation, and increased protein production to close the wound. Any interference with this process impairs tissue repair. Unfortunately, the treatment of malignancies requires the inhibition of migration, proliferation, and cellular metabolic activities. Many disease processes are treated with anti-inflammatory drugs. Therefore, any treatment with steroids,[37,38] chemotherapy agents,[39,40] or radiation[41,42] will impair the healing process. Surgeons must be aware that anyone treated with these agents has an increased risk of healing failure. This concept must be considered when treating patients with perioperative neoadjuvant therapy. The surgeon must optimize the patient's nutritional and metabolic status as much as possible before initiating multimodal cancer therapy. In addition, studies suggest that vitamin A may improve healing after radiation or steroid treatment.[17,18] Growth factors may also assist with improving tissue repair.[43–49]

BURNS IN THE ELDERLY

Burns can have a devastating effect on the elderly patient. First of all, more problems arise regarding healing of burn wounds in the elderly. In comparison with younger counterparts, minor burns are more likely to become full thickness because of thinner skin. With the decrease in the density of skin adnexa, especially hair follicles, the rate of re-epithelialization of superficial wounds is slower. It is well known that if a wound takes longer than 2 to 3 weeks to heal, there is an increased rate of hypertrophic scarring.[50] Therefore, fewer hair follicles mean that there is delayed healing and increased risks for excessive scar formation. A classic scenario is that an elderly person who lacks hair on his or her legs spills a hot liquid and sustains a superficial burn. Normally this burn would heal without problems but if there is a lack of hair follicles to initiate re-epithelialization, the wound fails to heal. These wounds are often described as "converting" to full thickness. In fact they did not convert but instead never had a chance to re-epithelialize. One advantage of being older is that as skin becomes looser, it has a better chance of contracting without producing tension. Because increased tension leads to more hypertrophic scarring, the patient with loose skin can contract a wound without producing a contracture.

The most important factor to be aware of in the elderly patient with a thermal injury is the increase in mortality. Major burns create tremendous metabolic stress for the patient. The systemic response to a burn includes an increased metabolic rate, increased protein breakdown, and greater exposure to infection. It is also clear that the elderly are less capable of handling the metabolic needs required to survive a major burn to the skin. The author likes to describe the problem as the following: to survive a burn, one must "run a marathon until they are healed." One can coerce a young person to handle the increased stress, but while the elderly attempt to deal with the metabolic demand, they soon tire and succumb to their injuries. This problem is manifest by the LA_{50} of a burn wound; that is, the size (total body surface area of the burn wound) of a thermal wound that leads to 50% mortality for the patient's age. The LA_{50} for a teenager is around 80%, meaning approximately half of teenagers with a burn wound to 80% of the skin will survive. The LA_{50} decreases with age so that an 80-year-old will have 50% mortality with an 8% burn wound. The reason for the increase in mortality with aging is not totally clear, but is likely related to the metabolic reserve of the organs as we age. In essence, the cells "run out of fuel" with increasing age. Just as athletes peak in the late teens and early twenties, the geriatric patient is less capable of producing the energy needed to meet the demands of a major injury. Lacking the ability to produce the supplies needed for healing the massive wound while at the same time being unable to meet the needs of organs leads to gradual loss of organ function, multiple organ dysfunction, and, eventually, death. Despite this problem, clinicians' ability to deal with the elderly has gradually improved over the years so that more elderly are surviving burns than ever before.

PROBLEM WOUNDS IN THE ELDERLY

Some chronic wounds are more common in the elderly population. These wounds are a significant burden to the population, and billions of dollars are spent every year to deal with such wounds. A basic knowledge of the pathophysiology and treatment of these wounds is essential to every clinician. The Wound Healing Society has provided excellent guidelines and references for dealing with the chronic, nonhealing ulcers.[51–56]

Pressure Ulcers

Pressure ulcers are very common wounds[51,52,57] that occur in approximately 10% of hospitalized patients. The cause of these ulcers is conceptually simple. Pressure greater than 30 mm Hg for prolonged periods leads to ischemia to the underlying tissues. Because pressure leads to pain, most people reposition themselves to avoid injury. Pressure ulcers tend to develop in those patients who have an inability to respond to pressure-related pain. Clearly a group at high risk for pressure-related wounds is patients with paraplegia or tetraplegia. The elderly are also at risk as they develop peripheral neuropathy. In addition, persons who are critically ill or immobile are at risk. As people, especially the elderly, lose fat or muscle mass, there is an increase in bony prominences. Pressure ulcers tend to occur at these sites: the presacral area, heels, and occipital scalp. In addition, incontinence leads to maceration and the increased risk of shear injuries, which can initiate skin loss leading to pressure ulcers.

Pressure ulcers are staged based on the depth of injury.[57,58] Stage 1 ulcers have intact but persistently reddened skin. Stage 2 ulcers have partial-thickness skin loss and thus have the potential for re-epithelialization with correction of the pressure exposure. Stage 3 ulcers are full thickness, and stage 4 ulcers have undermining and tunneling into the underlying tissues. The value of staging pressure ulcers has recently been challenged[59] but, clearly, the deeper the wound, the more the difficult the treatment of the wound. Prevention is the most important factor in reducing these problem wounds. The risk of a patient developing a pressure ulcer has been most commonly assessed using the Braden Score,[60] which is based on 6 factors: sensory perception, moisture, activity, mobility, nutrition, and friction/shear. Pressure ulcers have become an important issue for the government. The Center for Medicare and Medicaid Services (CMS) has considered pressure ulcers a "never event" and will levy fines of up to $10,000 if there is lack of monitoring and documentation for these wounds. Once a pressure ulcer develops it is difficult to treat. One must remove the source of pressure by moving the patient off the bony prominence. Several studies have documented improved healing using topical growth factors.[61,62] It is not uncommon to need a myocutaneous flap to cover the wound. Unfortunately, once a pressure ulcer develops, there is a high recurrence rate.

Arterial Insufficiency Ulcers

Peripheral vascular disease occurs in approximately 30% of persons older than 75 years, so it is an important issue for the elderly. Oxygen is required to heal any wound and, when it is lacking as a result of peripheral vascular disease, arterial ulcers develop.[53,54] A primary indication for the surgical repair of arterial insufficiency is a "limb at risk" with a nonhealing wound. Signs of vascular insufficiency include loss of pulse, loss of hair, dry and shiny skin, mummified toes, devitalized tissue with moist or dry crust, thickened toenails, cool skin, and purple skin with dependency. One should also check the ankle/brachial index, and more sophisticated vascular studies are usually indicated. Transcutaneous oxygen levels are helpful. If transcutaneous oxygen levels drop to less than 20 mm Hg, healing will not occur without revascularization. Prevention of these ulcers includes the usual methods of reducing atherosclerosis: cessation of smoking, treatment of hyperlipidemia, and exercise. Referral to a vascular surgeon is indicated to optimize conditions for wound healing. Once patients require revascularization, they have a 20% risk for developing another ulcer on the opposite limb.[63]

Venous Stasis Ulcers

Venous stasis ulcers are less of a problem for the elderly than they are for those who develop deep venous thrombosis.[55,56,64–67] In 1997, venous ulceration affected 2.5 million people with an estimated cost of $3 billion in the United States alone. Normally, muscular activity along with the venous valves directs the flow of blood back to the heart. After a deep vein thrombosis occurs, the valves in the central veins are often destroyed so that resulting venous valvular insufficiency leads to a direct column of blood from the heart to the foot. This increase in capillary hydrostatic pressure leads to leakage of serum to produce edema that decreases oxygen and nutrient delivery. There is deposition of fibrin, which acts as a "leukocyte trap" to produce chronic inflammation. The actual causes of these wounds are unknown, although many theories have been proposed.[68]

The classic venous stasis ulcer occurs above the medial malleolus, and is associated with edema and hyperpigmentation (lipodermatosclerosis). Once the ulcer develops it should be treated by reducing the venous hypertension and reducing edema, mainly be keeping the limb elevated. Pressure may also be reduced with pressure compression devices such as stockings or an Unna boot (fine mesh gauze with calamine lotion and zinc oxide applied with compression). Several studies have demonstrated the efficacy of using growth factors[69-71] or biological skin substitutes (which deliver growth factors).[72-75] The problem with these wounds is that the underlying defect, venous valvular insufficiency, is not resolved, so as soon as the person is upright the ulcers tend to recur. Methods for reducing venous backflow, such as subfascial endoscopic perforator surgery, may be helpful, but the real solution will be to recreate the venous valves. This solution as yet remains unresolved.

PREVENTION FOR THE ELDERLY

Prevention is the best way to reduce wound-healing problems in the elderly. It is interesting that simply teaching prevention is less effective than regulations that enforce prevention efforts. For instance, teaching someone to avoid placing gasoline on a fire does not prevent it from happening. People frequently practice risky behaviors or take shortcuts. Laws requiring smoke detectors in buildings, though resisted for years, have made a huge impact on fire-related deaths. It remains to be seen if the efforts of the CMS to make pressure ulcers a fineable "never event" may have some impact on the incidence of this complication. As the age and acuity of patients increase, it is likely that these chronic wounds will continue to occur.

The best way to prevent wounds in the elderly is to optimize their health. Optimal nutrition and avoidance of harmful habits such as smoking has already improved the survival of the elderly. Treatment of high cholesterol and hypertension will reduce atherosclerosis and peripheral vascular disease. Increased prophylaxis against venous thromboembolic disease should also reduce the risk of venous stasis ulcers. Aggressive treatment of diabetes mellitus along with aggressive management of its associated neuropathy should also reduce diabetic wound problems. Efforts to warn diabetic patients about the importance of monitoring their feet for signs of injury are also essential. There are many prevention aids available to reduce burn injuries. Lowering the water heater to around 50°C (120°F) will prevent scald injuries. Flame-retardant cigarettes extinguish themselves and thus do not set the furniture on fire. Making the elderly population aware that they no longer have the strength or reflexes they once had should also be helpful.

Fortunately, the geriatric population is taking better care of itself, as can be suggested by the increased numbers of aged living independently in society. More people are living into the nineties and hundreds than ever before. These persons are also in need of medical and surgical treatments that prolong their survival even further, so knowledge of their special healing problems is essential to all physicians who treat them.

REFERENCES

1. U.S. Census Bureau, Statistical Abstract of the United States: 2012. Available at: http://www.census.gov/compendia/statab/2012/tables/12s0009.pdf. Accessed June 28, 2012.
2. Gosain A, DiPietro LA. Aging and wound healing. World J Surg 2004;28:321-6.
3. Zouboulis CC, Makrantonaki E. Clinical aspects and molecular diagnostics of skin aging. Clin Dermatol 2011;29:3-14.
4. Ramos-e-Silva M, Boza JC, Cestari TF. Effects of age (neonates and elderly) on skin barrier function. Clin Dermatol 2012;30:274-6.
5. Wulf HC, Sandby-Moller J, Kobayasi T, et al. Skin aging and natural photoprotection. Micron 2004;35:185-91.

6. Birch MP, Messenger JF, Messenger AG. Hair density, hair diameter and the prevalence of female pattern hair loss. Br J Dermatol 2001;144:297–304.

7. Sharma R. Skin age testing criteria: characterization of human skin structures by 500 MHz MRI multiple contrast and image processing. Phys Med Biol 2010;55: 3959–79.

8. Greenhalgh DG. Wound healing. Chapter 46. In: Herndon D, editor. Total burn care. 3rd edition. Philadelphia: Saunders Elsevier, Inc; 2007. p. 578–95.

9. Sussman MD. Aging of connective tissue: physiologic properties of healing wounds in young and old rats. Am J Physiol 1973;224:1167–71.

10. Guergova S, Dufour A. Thermal sensitivity in the elderly: a review. Ageing Res Rev 2011;10:80–92.

11. Howes EL, Briggs H, Shea R. Effect of complete and partial starvation on the rate of fibroplasia in the healing wound. Arch Surg 1933;26:846–58.

12. Rhoads JE, Fliegelman MT, Panzer LM. The mechanism of delayed wound healing in the presence of hypoproteinemia. JAMA 1942;118:21–5.

13. Daly JM, Vars HM, Dudvich SJ. Effects of protein depletion on strength of colonic anastomoses. Surg Gynecol Obstet 1972;134:15–21.

14. Irvin TT. Effects of malnutrition and hyperalimentation on wound healing. Surg Gynecol Obstet 1978;146:33–7.

15. Greenhalgh DG, Gamelli RL. Immunomodulators and wound healing. J Trauma 1987;27:510–4.

16. Bartlett MK, Jones CM, Ryan AE. Vitamin C and wound healing. I. Experimental wounds in guinea pigs. N Engl J Med 1942;226:469–73.

17. Ehrlich HP, Hunt TK. Effects of cortisone and vitamin A on wound healing. Ann Surg 1968;167:324–8.

18. Levenson SM, Gruber CA, Rettura G, et al. Supplemental vitamin A prevents the acute radiation-induced defect in wound healing. Ann Surg 1984;200:494–512.

19. Pories WJ. Acceleration of healing with zinc oxide. Ann Surg 1967;165:432–6.

20. Pinnell SR, Martin GR. The cross linking of collagen and elastin. Proc Natl Acad Sci U S A 1968;61:708–14.

21. Liusuwan RA, Palmieri T, Warden N, et al. Impaired healing due to copper deficiency in a pediatric burn: a case report. J Trauma 2006;51:464–6.

22. Seifter E, Rettura G, Barbul A, et al. Arginine: an essential amino acid for injured rats. Surgery 1978;84:224–30.

23. McMurry JF Jr. Wound healing with diabetes mellitus. Surg Clin North Am 1984; 64:769–78.

24. Goodson WH III, Hunt TK. Wound healing and the diabetic patient. Surg Gynecol Obstet 1979;149:600–8.

25. Greenhalgh DG. Wound healing and diabetes mellitus. Clin Plast Surg 2003;30: 37–45.

26. Margolis DJ, Kantor J, Berlin JA. Healing of diabetic neuropathic foot ulcers receiving standard treatment. A meta-analysis. Diabetes Care 1999;22:692–5.

27. Yue DK, McLennan S, Marsh M, et al. Effects of experimental diabetes, uremia, and malnutrition on wound healing. Diabetes 1987;36:295–9.

28. Barsun A, Sen S, Palmieri TL, et al. A ten year review of lower extremity burns in diabetics: small burns that lead to major problems. J Burn Care Res 2013;34(2): 255–60.

29. Kamal K, Powell RJ, Sumpio BE. The pathobiology of diabetes mellitus: implications for surgeons. J Am Coll Surg 1996;183:271–89.

30. Medzhitov R. Origin and physiological roles of inflammation. Nature 2008;454: 428–35.

31. Steed DL, Attinger C, Colaizzi T, et al. Guidelines for the treatment of diabetic ulcers. Wound Repair Regen 2006;14:680–92.
32. Steed DL, Attinger C, Brem H, et al. Guidelines for the prevention of diabetic ulcers. Wound Repair Regen 2008;16:169–74.
33. Armstrong DG, Nguyen HC, Lavery LA, et al. Off-loading the diabetic foot: a randomized clinical trial. Diabetes Care 2001;24:1019–22.
34. Steed DL, The Diabetic Ulcer Study Group. Clinical evaluation of recombinant human platelet-derived growth factor for the treatment of lower extremity diabetic ulcers. J Vasc Surg 1995;21:71–81.
35. Embil JM, Papp K, Sibbald G, et al. Recombinant human platelet-derived growth factor-BB (becaplermin) for healing chronic lower extremity diabetic ulcers: an open-label clinical evaluation of efficacy. Wound Repair Regen 2000;8:162–8.
36. Veves A, Falanga V, Armstrong DG, et al. Graftskin, a human skin equivalent, is effective in the management of noninfected neuropathic diabetic foot ulcers: a prospective, randomized multicenter clinical trial. Diabetes Care 2001;24:290–5.
37. Howes EL, Plotz CM, Blunt JW, et al. Retardation of wound healing by cortisone. Surgery 1950;28:177–81.
38. Sandberg N. Time relationship between administration of cortisone and wound healing in rats. Acta Chir Scand 1964;127:446–55.
39. Ferguson MK. The effects of antineoplastic agents on wound healing. Surg Gynecol Obstet 1982;154:421–9.
40. Falcone RE, Napp JF. Chemotherapy and wound healing. Surg Clin North Am 1984;64:779–95.
41. Reinisch JF, Puckett CL. Management of radiation wounds. Surg Clin North Am 1984;64:795–802.
42. Luce EA. The irradiated wound. Surg Clin North Am 1984;64:821–9.
43. Laato M, Heino J, Kahari VM, et al. Epidermal growth factor (EGF) prevents methylprednisolone-induced inhibition of wound healing. J Surg Res 1989;47:354–9.
44. Pierce GF, Mustoe TA, Lingelbach J, et al. Transforming growth factor β reverses the glucocorticoid-induced wound healing deficit in rats: possible regulation in macrophages by platelet-derived growth factor. Proc Natl Acad Sci U S A 1989;86:2229–33.
45. Beck LS, DeGuzman L, Lee WP, et al. TGF-β1 accelerates wound healing: reversal of steroid-impaired healing in rats and rabbits. Growth Factors 1991;5:295–300.
46. Lawrence WT, Sporn MB, Gorschboth C, et al. The reversal of an adriamycin induced healing impairment with chemoattractants and growth factors. Ann Surg 1986;203:142–7.
47. Mustoe TA, Purdy J, Gramates P, et al. Reversal of impaired wound healing in irradiated rats by platelet-derived growth factor-BB. Am J Surg 1989;158:345–50.
48. Bernstein EF, Harisiadis L, Saloman G, et al. Transforming growth factor beta improves healing of radiation-impaired wounds. J Invest Dermatol 1991;97:430–4.
49. Tattini C, Manchio J, Zaporojan V, et al. The role of TGF-β and FGF in the treatment of radiation-induced wounds using a novel drug delivery system. Plast Reconstr Surg 2008;122:1036–45.
50. Deitch EA, Wheelahan TM, Rose MP, et al. Hypertrophic scars: analysis of variables. J Trauma 1983;23:895–8.
51. Whitney J, Phillips L, Aslam R, et al. Guidelines for the treatment of pressure ulcers. Wound Repair Regen 2006;14:663–79.

52. Stechmiller JK, Cowan L, Whitney J, et al. Guidelines for the prevention of pressure ulcers. Wound Repair Regen 2008;16:151–68.
53. Hopf HW, Ueno C, Aslam R, et al. Guidelines for the treatment of arterial insufficiency ulcers. Wound Repair Regen 2006;14:693–710.
54. Hopf HW, Ueno C, Aslam R, et al. Guidelines for the prevention of arterial insufficiency ulcers. Wound Repair Regen 2008;16:175–88.
55. Robson MC, Cooper DM, Aslam R, et al. Guidelines for the treatment of venous ulcers. Wound Repair Regen 2006;14:649–62.
56. Robson MC, Cooper DM, Aslam R, et al. Guidelines for the prevention of venous ulcers. Wound Repair Regen 2008;16:147–50.
57. Lyder CH. Pressure ulcer prevention and management. JAMA 2003;289:223–6.
58. Bluestein D, Javaheri A. Pressure ulcers: prevention, evaluation, and management. Am Fam Physician 2008;78:1186–94.
59. Sibbald RG, Krasner DL, Woo KY. Pressure ulcer staging revisited: superficial skin changes & deep pressure ulcer framework. Adv Skin Wound Care 2011;24:571–80.
60. Braden BJ, Bergstrom NA. Clinical utility of the Braden Scale for predicting pressure sore risk. Decubitus 1989;2:44–51.
61. Mustoe TA, Cutler NR, Allman RM, et al. A phase II study to evaluate recombinant platelet-derived growth factor-BB in the treatment of stage 3 and 4 pressure ulcers. Arch Surg 1994;129:213–9.
62. Rees RS, Robson MC, Smiell JM, et al. Becaplermin gel in the treatment of pressure ulcers: a phase II randomized double-blind, placebo-controlled study. Wound Repair Regen 1999;7:141–7.
63. Tarry WC, Walsh DB, Birkmeyer NJ, et al. Fate of contralateral leg after infrainguinal bypass. J Vasc Surg 1998;27:1039–48.
64. Gillespie DL. Venous ulcer diagnosis, treatment, and prevention of recurrences. J Vasc Surg 2010;52:8S–14S.
65. Robertson LE, Fowkes F. Epidemiology of chronic venous disease. Phlebology 2008;23:103–11.
66. Ruckley CV. Socioeconomic impact of chronic venous insufficiency and leg ulcers. Angiology 1997;48:67–9.
67. Van den Oever RH, Debbaut B, Simon I. Socio-economic impact of chronic venous insufficiency: an underestimated public health problem. Int Angiol 1998;17:161–7.
68. Liu YC, Margolis DJ, Isseroff RR. Does inflammation have a role in the pathogenesis of venous ulcers? A critical review of the evidence. J Invest Dermatol 2011;131:818–27.
69. DaCosta RM, Ribeiro J, Aniceto C, et al. Randomized, double-blind, placebo-controlled, dose-ranging study of granulocyte-macrophage colony-stimulating factor in patients with chronic venous ulcers. Wound Repair Regen 1999;7:17–25.
70. Falanga V, Eaglstein WH, Bucalo B, et al. Topical use of human recombinant epidermal growth factor (h-EGF) in venous ulcers. J Dermatol Surg Oncol 1992;18:604–6.
71. Robson MC, Phillips LG, Cooper DM, et al. The safety and effect of transforming growth factor-B2 for treatment of venous stasis ulcers. Wound Repair Regen 1995;3:157–67.
72. Falanga V, Margolis D, Alvarez O, et al. Rapid healing of venous ulcers and the lack of clinical rejection with an allogeneic cultured human skin equivalent. Human Skin Equivalent Investigators Group. Arch Dermatol 1998;134:293–300.
73. Atillasoy E. The safety and efficacy of Graftskin (Apligraf) in the treatment of venous leg ulcers: a multicenter, randomized, controlled clinical trial. Wounds 2000;12(Suppl A):20A–6A.

74. Pierik EG, vanUrk H, Hop WC, et al. Endoscopic versus open subfascial division of incompetent perforating veins in the treatment of venous leg ulceration: a randomized trial. J Vasc Surg 1997;26:1049–54.

75. Sybrandy JE, vanGent WB, Pierik EG, et al. Endoscopic versus open subfascial division of incompetent perforating veins in the treatment of venous leg ulceration: long-term follow-up. J Vasc Surg 2001;33:1028–32.

Management of Fractures in a Geriatric Surgical Patient

Jide Tinubu, MD, Thomas M. Scalea, MD*

KEYWORDS

- Geriatric fractures • Early fracture fixation • Hip fractures
- Vertebral compression fractures • Lateral compression pelvic fractures

KEY POINTS

- Joint replacement surgery has increased mobility in older patients.
- Elderly patients are no longer confined to a life of inactivity; however, they are more likely to become injured and present to trauma centers for care.
- Bone aging puts the elderly patient at high risk for fractures when they are injured.
- It is important to assess adequacy of cardiovascular function in all geriatric trauma patients, particularly those with fractures.
- Lateral compression fractures are the most common injury mechanism in older patients.

INTRODUCTION

Trauma is becoming an increasingly common problem in geriatric patients, and fractures are a frequent injury sustained by the elderly. Life expectancy continues to rise. Recent advances in medical care for common problems, such as heart disease and diabetes, have allowed people to live longer and better lives. For instance, calcium channel blockers and β-blockers, medications that are part of everyday practice, have only existed for 30 years. Surgical advances, such as percutaneous treatment for coronary artery disease, as well as the recognition that coronary bypass grafting can be safely performed in elderly patients, have allowed older patients to be more active without symptoms such as chest pain or shortness of breath. Joint replacement surgery has increased mobility in older patients. Thus, elderly patients are no longer confined to a life of inactivity. They are out of their homes and interacting in the community, exercising and leading active lives. Thus, they are more likely to become injured and present to trauma centers for care.

There are several factors that predispose elderly individuals to trauma, including poor vision and slowed reflexes.[1,2] Trauma is potentially devastating to the elderly

R Adams Cowley Shock Trauma Center, Department of Orthopedics, University of Maryland School of Medicine, 22 South Greene Street, Baltimore, MD 21201, USA
* Corresponding author.
E-mail address: tscalea@umm.edu

Surg Clin N Am 95 (2015) 115–128
http://dx.doi.org/10.1016/j.suc.2014.09.017
0039-6109/15/$ – see front matter © 2015 Elsevier Inc. All rights reserved.
surgical.theclinics.com

population owing to poor physiologic reserves and higher incidence of comorbid conditions.[3] Relatively low-energy forces can result in major injuries owing to the decreased bone density seen with osteoporosis and atrophic soft tissues.[4] These common risk factors result in recognizable patterns of bony injuries. Fractures of the hip, spine, proximal humerus, and wrist are disproportionately represented in the advanced age group.[5–7] Any one of the fractures can be a life-changing event and result in a previously independent individual falling into a pattern of hospitalization, rapid deconditioning, and generalized decline.

Bone aging, described in more detail elsewhere in this article, put the elderly patient at very high risk for fractures when they are injured. Although polytrauma fractures are present in virtually every elderly patient who is badly injured, isolated fractures from a relatively low-energy mechanism are far more common. As trauma care becomes increasingly regionalized, older patients with significant comorbidities are increasingly being referred to trauma centers. These patients are almost always admitted to the general surgery trauma service, not to the orthopedic service. Thus, it is important for general surgeons to be conversant with the issues around fracture care in the elderly. For instance, at the R Adams Cowley Shock Trauma Center last year, we admitted 6158 patients from the scene or as transfers, 1955 of whom (32%) had extremity fractures. Approximately 1300 of these patients were over the age of 65, and 426 (34%) of them sustained extremity fractures.

GENERAL APPROACH TO THE TRAUMA PATIENT WITH FRACTURES

The initial evaluation of the older patient with fractures is not different from any other trauma patient. Like younger patients, older patients are at risk for serious injury within the head, chest, abdomen, and retroperitoneum. These injuries take priority over fractures and must be addressed first. Initial care of the fractures should be to stop external hemorrhage and to perform fracture reduction when feasible. Perfusion distal to the fracture should be assessed by physical examination and/or studies such as duplex ultrasonography, compute tomographic angiography, or a catheter study.

Injury burden is magnified by presence of fractures, but the cardiovascular response to injury in older patients is blunted. Over 20 years ago, Scalea and colleagues[8] demonstrated that early invasive monitoring in high-risk polytrauma geriatric patients was associated with improved survival. In that study, patients commonly had nonhypotensive cardiogenic shock that was not recognized by measuring blood pressure, pulse rate, or urine output. Assessment with a pulmonary artery catheter was necessary to make early diagnosis and direct therapy. Philosophically, this is similar to the early goal-directed therapy described by Rivers and colleagues[9] for septic shock, a treatment strategy practiced every day. The presence of more than 1 long bone fracture places geriatric patients in the high-risk group. Thus, it is important to understand that fractures by themselves are a cardiovascular stressor. Although pulmonary artery catheters are no longer used commonly, it remains important to assess the adequacy of cardiovascular function in all geriatric trauma patients, particularly those with fractures.

SKELETAL CHANGES WITH AGING

The bony skeleton is a biologically active organ system that serves many functions. First, it provides a rigid framework for support and attachment of muscles that allow for efficient movement. Vital organs are afforded protection by bones. Bone marrow contains stem cells and actively produces multiple blood cells. The skeleton represent the body's largest store of calcium, which and is acted upon by the endocrine system to regulate serum calcium levels within narrow ranges, vital for many cellular functions.

Bone is composed of both an inorganic and an organic phase, with the mineral content of bone making up about 60% of its dry weight.[10] The majority of the mineral content of bone is in the form of calcium hydroxyapatite. The organic component of bone is composed largely of type I collagen. Both the organic and inorganic components of bone are acted upon by the specialized cells dispersed throughout its structure. Osteoblasts promote formation of bone by secreting type I collagen that is later mineralized. Osteoclasts are responsible for resorption of bone. Osteocytes form the majority of cells within bone and are active in maintaining serum calcium and phosphorus concentrations. All of these cells have receptors that respond to signal from the endocrine system as well as electrical and physical stimuli and thereby regulate bone density and serum mineral concentrations.

During the first 3 decades of life, the skeleton progressively increases in mineral content and bone mass, usually peaking in the third decade.[11] The ultimate bone mass achieved is largely determined by hereditary factors, but can also be affected by dietary habits. Thereafter, there is a gradual decline in bone mass. The rate of loss increases after age 50 and is significantly greater among women.[12] It is accelerated in many disease states, and responsive to activity level.[13–15]

A gross cross-section of bone shows that it is not a homogenous structure. The outer layer of bone, called the cortex, is densely packed and organized into layers called lamellae. The inner medullary cavity is much more porous and has a spongy appearance, referred to as trabecular or cancellous bone. The outer cortex provides much of the strength of bone and the medullary canal allows space for hematopoiesis and storage of fat. The overall architecture of bone is specialized for its weight-bearing function. The central tubular section of long bones, called the diaphysis, is dominated by thick cortex and relatively narrow medullary canal. This gives a great deal of strength to resist axial load and bending stress. Toward their ends, long bones widen or flare into a metaphysis. Here, trabecular bone dominates and more efficiently distributes forces transmitted across joints.

Bone is generally well-vascularized, receiving its blood supply from multiple sources, including:

1. Dedicated vessels that usually pierce long bones in the diaphyseal section and transmit blood from central to peripheral;
2. Tendon/ligament attachments near the ends of bones (peripheral to central direction); and
3. Periosteum/muscle via small perforators.

These multiple blood supplies provide a certain level of redundancy and bone has a remarkable ability to retain viability as long as some blood supply remains intact. Adequate blood supply is critical to the proper function and healing of bone and is often at risk with severely traumatized limbs.

Bone Changes in Older Age

Bone changes occur during normal aging in both men and women. Changes are both quantitative and qualitative in nature. Decreasing levels of naturally occurring anabolic steroids result in gradual demineralization of bone. Decreased physical activity and dietary inadequacies common in the elderly population tend to exacerbate the progressive loss of bone. Bone tissue is particularly responsive to mechanical loading, and the magnitude of bone mass loss as a consequence of decreased physical activity may not be fully appreciated.[16]

Decreased mineralization of bone, termed relative osteopenia, is readily discernible on plain radiographs, but a diagnosis of osteoporosis has specific criteria. Risk factors for osteoporosis include advanced age, low body mass index, lack of impact activities, and female gender, but it must be stressed that anyone can be affected. Osteoporosis is not considered a normal progression of aging, but is in fact a pathologic condition where normal physiologic loads can result in fractures. The diagnosis of osteoporosis is made using a specific set of criteria comparing the bone mineral density of a patient to an average young healthy individual.[17] Relative osteopenia (decreased bone density) is readily identified on plain radiographs and no specific diagnostic criteria are needed.

In addition to the changes in bone density, there is a progressive change in the architecture of bone with aging. Bone from healthy, older individuals when compared with younger samples is larger in overall diameter but with a thinner, weaker outer cortex; a greater proportion of cancellous bone; lesser hematopoietic activity; and greater brittleness. These changes are magnified in the presence of many disease states, including kidney disease, diabetes, and liver disease.

Regardless of whether the bony changes result from normal physiologic aging or an underlying medical condition, the resulting bone is less capable of dealing with physical stress. Exposure to trauma results in fractures and the weakened bone challenges our ability to treat them using conventional methods.

FRACTURES IN THE ELDERLY PATIENT
Low Energy

Fractures that result from relatively low-energy injuries, such as fall from standing, are considered fragility fractures (**Fig. 1**). Vertebral compression fractures, distal radius fractures, and fractures around the hip are common in the elderly population and have been used as a marker for identifying individuals with osteoporosis and therefore at increased risk for fractures in the future.[5–7] Proximal humerus fractures and ankle fractures also commonly fall under this category. Any individual with a fragility fracture should be identified for possible treatment of their underlying osteopenia, which has been shown to decrease the incidence of secondary fractures.

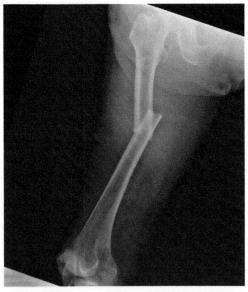

Fig. 1. Midshaft femur fracture in older patient caused by a ground-level fall.

High Energy

Although low-energy fractures are far more common in the elderly patients, high-energy fractures do occur. The energy imparted to weakened bone produces fractures of increased severity and complexity. The level of energy imparted during an injury is directly related to the level of comminution of a fracture, as well as the number and size of fracture fragments produced when a bone is broken. Higher energy injuries have an increased number of fracture fragments. Fracture patterns with increased comminution have less inherent stability in an injured limb.

With any fracture, there is always some degree of soft tissue injury. Higher energy fractures are associated with greater injury to the surrounding soft tissues. In the elderly population, the surrounding skin, muscle, and tendons are often attenuated and thus more susceptible to injury. Disruption of these structures compromises the successful treatment of fractures, which are dependent on the blood supply delivered to bone to heal. Open fractures increase the risk of infection and contribute to blood loss. In addition to local tissue disruption, high-energy mechanisms often produce injuries to multiple organ systems and multiple fractured limbs.

RATIONALE FOR TREATMENT

The approach to treatment of fractures in the elderly population is altered based on their particular needs. In younger, active patients an intra-articular fracture may be aggressively treated in an effort to avoid posttraumatic arthritis and preserve the native articular surface joint. This approach often involves prolonged surgical procedures and periods of limited weight bearing postoperatively. This approach may not be best in older individuals in whom it may be advisable to minimize physiologic insult associated with surgery. It is best for elderly patients to be mobilized as early as possible, because their function tends to deteriorate significantly with immobilization. A good example of this is a femoral neck fracture. Although less common in the younger population, when it does occur, the accepted approach is to preserve the native hip and fix the fracture anatomically. In contrast, in the geriatric population, arthroplasty is the better approach because this allows the patient to mobilize and bear weight immediately, minimizing morbidity and mortality. Similar approaches have been used in patients with severely comminuted fractures of the proximal humerus and distal femur.

A patient's level of function before injury also influences the decision on how to treat a fracture. It is obviously unwise to expose a patient who does not ambulate to the risk of a major surgical procedure to achieve a perfect reduction. In addition, it is common for an elderly patient to decrease their level of ambulatory function after a fracture, even if it is treated well and heals uneventfully. Patients and family members need to be aware of this and prepared for adjustments before patient transition back to the home environment. Previously independent individuals may now need substantial help and may no longer be able to live independently. The overriding principle is to focus efforts on returning patients to their expected level of function as soon as possible, to prevent progressive decline and minimize the impact of injuries on quality of life.

TIMING OF FRACTURE FIXATION

Our understanding of the optimal timing for fracture fixation has evolved over years. In 1985, Seibel and colleagues,[18] demonstrated that fracture fixation within 24 hours in patients with femur fractures was associated with significantly fewer complications and a lesser mortality rate. Thus, early fracture fixation became the norm, particularly in polytrauma patients. However, later data questioned whether early fracture fixation was necessary, suggesting that outcome was more closely related to the actual injuries, rather than the timing of the fixation. Finally, several articles suggested that early fracture fixation may be deleterious in certain groups, particularly those with brain injury. Other studies, however, did not confirm those initial concerns.[19–21]

There are a number of reasons why early fracture fixation in elderly patients would be ideal. Patients with fractures often remain in bed, sometimes in skeletal traction until surgical stabilization. Early fracture fixation mobilizes them out of bed, allowing the chest to get upright and increasing pulmonary function. Elderly patients have increased ventilation perfusion mismatch at rest. Particularly if they have rib fractures, they are especially prone to developing atelectasis. The hypoxia that accompanies this may require mechanical ventilation, increasing the risk of ventilator-associated pneumonia.

It is difficult to prevent pressure sores in patients in bed with fractures that have not yet been stabilized. Skin changes associated with aging make skin breakdown more common, placing the elderly person at particular risk for pressure ulceration of the skin. Narcotic analgesics come with particular risks in elderly patients. Mental confusion, acute delirium, and gastrointestinal side effects all accompany the use of narcotics. Simply taking the elderly patient out of their environment and placing them in the hospital disrupts their sleep–wake cycle, causing confusion, delirium, or both. The hospital environment does not allow for normal activity schedules, making proper sleep problematic. Disruption of the patient's normal sleep cycle is also associated with confusion. These symptoms are commonly treated with other medications, often sedatives, all of which have their own set of side effects. Thus, the safest thing for an elderly patient is to rapidly receive care and be discharged out of the inpatient environment as soon as possible.

The decision regarding the timing of optimal fracture fixation in older patients is a discussion about risks and benefits (**Table 1**). All too often, the knee jerk response is to simply obtain a medical or cardiology consultation for "clearance." Typically, this delays care. If a patient is admitted in the evening or at night, these consultations rarely take place until the next day. Virtually always, the consultants request previous medical records and then order a battery of tests, usually an electrocardiograph, additional laboratory tests, and an echocardiogram. These tests are often not done until the following day and then the consultant must review the results before making recommendations. Thus, fracture therapy is delayed 48 hours or even longer to obtain the "clearance" that was requested.

Rational decision making requires consideration of a number of issues. The first question involves assessing the physiologic stress of the surgery being planned. For

| Table 1 | |
| Preoperative evaluation | |
Examination	Role in Preoperative Pharmacy
Chest x-ray	Diagnoses acute and chronic pulmonary pathology
Electrocardiograph	Diagnoses acute cardiac pathology, ventricular hypertrophy and remote myocardial infarction
Echocardiogram	Determines cardiac (valvular) problems and ventricular performers at rest
Nuclear medicine stress test	Determine cardiac function with stress and presence of reversible ischemia
Cardiac catheterization	Identifies structural coronary artery abnormalities

instance, fixation of a radius fracture is a relatively small operation with virtually no soft tissue injury and minimal blood loss. Intramedullary nailing of a femur is associated with far more blood loss and tissue damage. Thus, this procedure entails a much more substantial cardiovascular stress.

One must then assess the ability of the patient to withstand the stress necessary to undergo fracture fixation. Taking a good history provides the most important information. Patients should be assessed for exercise tolerance. It is important to be particularly specific with these questions. Elderly patients with coronary disease may limit their exercise to avoid having angina. Patients with arthritis or peripheral vascular disease may be unable to exercise sufficiently to have symptoms of coronary disease manifest. Thus, specific questions such as, "if I put you out on the street on a nice spring day, how far could you walk?" or "Can you climb a flight of stairs?" are far better than asking if patients if they experience chest pain when walking.

Physical examination should be directed at identifying potentially correctable structural cardiovascular pathology. Conditions such as critical valvular disease should be identifiable by auscultation of the heart. Significant peripheral edema or ascites may suggest heart failure. The electrocardiogram should be scrutinized for signs of left ventricular hypertrophy or a previous myocardial infarction. Patient medications should be carefully reviewed. Often, patients do not remember all of their medical problems. Reviewing medications may give some clue as to conditions for which they are receiving treatment. A short discussion with the patient's primary care doctor can be invaluable, such as getting an accurate medication list, results from previous testing, and a baseline electrocardiograph.

One should then discuss options with the orthopedic surgeon or whoever else will be performing the operation. Issues like anticipated blood loss, whether a lesser operation would be acceptable, and/or whether a nonoperative option exists need to be discussed to make a rational decision. For instance, a patient with a fracture of a weight-bearing bone in the lower extremity, such as a femur fracture or a hip fracture, likely has no nonoperative option. Thus, delaying surgery makes little sense. On the other hand, a patient with an odontoid fracture may be able to be treated for a period of time, or even definitively, with a cervical collar. Although the cervical collar may not be ideal therapy, it may be acceptable therapy in patients who are extremely high risk.

Diagnostic testing should be undertaken to answer specific questions and concerns. Blanket application of a battery of tests makes little sense. An echocardiogram measures ventricular function and valvular anatomy. It is unable to predict how the heart will respond to stresses during surgery. An electrocardiograph and cardiac enzymes can identify patients who are having acute ischemic events. However, they do not predict outcome after surgery. Thus, in elderly patients with good exercise tolerance, no history of heart disease, and a normal physical examination, who has a fracture that has no nonoperative options, the decision to proceed with surgery is unlikely to be altered by a series of tests.

If one wishes to assess how the patient's heart will respond to stresses of surgery, either a dobutamine echocardiogram or a nuclear medicine stress test needs to be ordered. These are only valuable in high-risk patients and clinicians should order them only if there is a significant chance that they will change outcome.

The timing of surgery in hip fractures has been extensively reviewed. The data suggest that early fixation is ideal. Lefaivre and colleagues[22] reviewed 607 patients with hip fractures treated at Vancouver General Hospital. Delay of surgery, comorbidities, age, and type of fracture all significantly increased time to discharge. Clearly, the only modifiable variable here is the delay of surgery. A delay of longer than 24 hours from the time of admission to operative fixation was also a significant predictor of minor complications. A delay of longer than 48 hours was associated with an increased risk of major medical complications and pressure sores. Simunovic and colleagues[23] reviewed 16 observational studies on hip fractures, which included approximately 13,500 patients. This demonstrated that earlier operative intervention was associated with a significant reduction in mortality. Earlier surgery also reduced the rate of pneumonia and pressure sores. Moja and colleagues[24] performed a meta-analysis of more than 190,000 patients with hip fractures. Early hip surgery reduced the risk of death, as well as pressure sores. Finally, Leung and colleagues[25] also performed a literature review, concluding that there was widespread evidence that morbidity, the incidence of pressure sores, and hospital stay was improved by early surgical therapy. They concluded that it is beneficial for elderly patients to have operative fixation as soon as they met basic anesthetic requirements.

Hip fractures are clearly the type of fractures that have been studied the most often. However, it seems reasonable to think that other fractures, particularly lower extremity fractures, would behave similarly. Thus, an attempt should be made to optimize patients as early as possible and proceed with operative fixation within 24 hours if possible, unless there are significant contraindications to fracture fixation.

COMMON FRACTURES IN THE ELDERLY TRAUMA PATIENT
Hip Fractures

Fractures around the hip are divided into 2 main categories based on the location of the fracture line in relation to the hip joint capsule. Femoral neck fractures are within the joint capsule, and together they account for a significant number of injuries in the elderly population. These are usually the result of low-energy trauma.

Femoral neck fracture is what we traditionally think of as a hip fracture (**Figs. 2 and 3**). When displaced, blood supply to the femoral head is often completely disrupted. Because of this, attempts to preserve the native hip often result in failure owing avascular necrosis, nonunion, or late displacement of fractures despite fixation. Hemiarthroplasty (femoral head replacement) allows for immediate mobilization and full weight bearing. A total hip arthroplasty provides durable, long-lasting solution for more active individuals, whereas hemiarthroplasty is a less invasive procedure suitable for people with low physical demands (**Figs. 4 and 5**).

Intertrochanteric fractures usually do not disrupt blood supply and reliably heal when fixed appropriately. Arthroplasty is therefore not indicated. Implants and techniques have been developed over time that allow immediate weight bearing.

Upper extremity fractures

Upper extremity injuries may not compromise mobility in the average person. However, an older patient who relies on support devices such as walkers for ambulation can be significantly disabled by even an isolated upper extremity fracture. This is especially true when combined with injuries to other extremities.

Distal radius fractures present a wide range of injury severity from minimally displaced fractures treated nonoperatively to completely unstable open injuries. Overall strategy involves tailoring treatment to the specific needs of the patient. Low-demand patients tolerate the decreased range of motion associated with nonoperative treatment of these injuries well. Individuals who require a high degree of manual dexterity for work or pleasure activities may benefit from anatomic reduction and rigid internal fixation, which allows for earlier joint range of motion and potentially decreased joint stiffness. Proximal humerus fractures often do well with nonoperative treatment. Management is largely centered around pain control by minimizing motion at the fracture site.

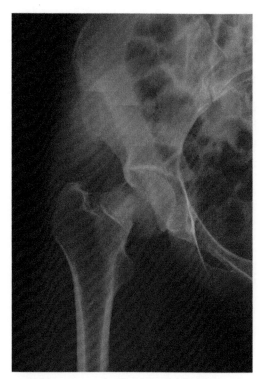

Fig. 2. Hip fracture treated by open reduction internal fixation.

Ankle Fractures

Ankle injuries in general are very common and this holds true in the older population as well. Owing to the exposure of the lower extremities and the relative paucity of soft tissue coverage in the distal lower extremity, open fractures are commonly encountered around the ankle. Displaced fracture fragments in closed fractures can lacerate skin if extremities are not adequately immobilized and very rapidly lead to pressure necrosis of overlying skin if not promptly reduced. Attenuated soft tissue envelope in older patients must be managed. Peripheral vascular disease and chronic edema further

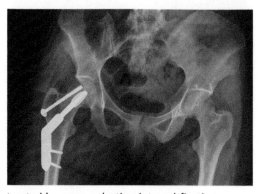

Fig. 3. Hip fracture treated by open reduction internal fixation.

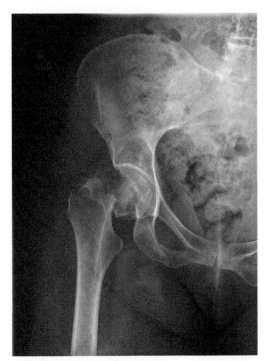

Fig. 4. Hip fracture treated by total hip arthroplasty.

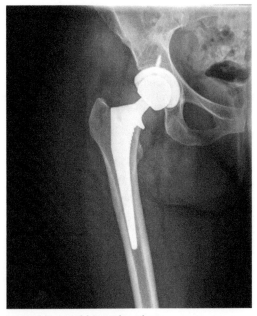

Fig. 5. Hip fracture treated by total hip arthroplasty.

complicate the management of ankle fractures, with an increased risk of infection, delayed healing, and often severely osteopenic bone.

Periprosthetic Fractures

A periprosthetic fracture is a broken bone that occurs around previously implanted orthopedic hardware (**Fig. 6**). Most commonly this involves the components of a total hip or knee replacement. It is a serious complication that most often requires surgery. These fractures are rare; however, because more patients are undergoing hip replacement surgery, the number of periprosthetic fractures is expected to increase (www.aaos.org). A major consideration for management is whether or not implants remain well fixed to bone after a fracture. Well-fixed implants can usually remain in place while the fracture is stabilized with new hardware. If implants are dislodged from the bone or loosened, treatment usually involves revision by a total joint specialist.

Pelvic Fractures

In younger people, pelvic fractures are a marker of injury severity, because it takes a great deal of force to fracture the boney pelvis. The same is not true in elderly patients, in whom pelvic fractures may occur after relatively minimal trauma, such as falling from standing or from a chair. Like pelvic fractures in the younger patients, however, pelvic fractures in the elderly may represent a source of substantial hemorrhage. Even an isolated pelvic fracture in an older person can be a life-threatening injury.

Initial resuscitation principles for pelvic fractures are the same in older people as they are in younger people.[26]

In anterior posterior compression fractures, the widening of the pelvis often injures major branches of the hypogastric artery. However, in lateral compression fractures, the pelvic implodes, it does not explode. Therefore, hemorrhage is far less common.

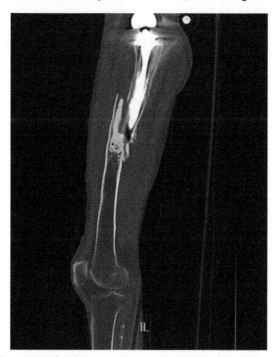

Fig. 6. Computed tomography demonstrating periprosthetic femur fracture.

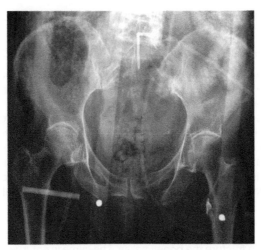

Fig. 7. Lateral compression pelvic fracture in older patient hit by a car.

In older patients, however, it is likely that the smaller blood vessels in the posterior pelvis cannot develop vasospasm, as they commonly do in younger patients. The lack of soft tissue turgor as one ages limits the ability to tamponade hemorrhage from these seemingly small blood vessels. Thus, hemorrhage is very common in older patients who sustain lateral compression.

Lateral compression fractures are by far the most common injury mechanism in older patients. In younger patients, lateral compression fractures are the least common source of substantial hemorrhage. Anterior posterior compression fractures bleed more often. However, in older patients, lateral compression fractures are common sources of hemorrhage. Initial methods of hemostasis, other than resuscitation and transfusion, involve reducing the bony elements of the pelvis. This maneuver is designed to limit the pelvic volume, thereby providing tamponade for venous hemorrhage. Reducing the fracture fragments likely also reduces blood loss from the fracture fragments themselves. In anterior posterior compression fractures, this is easily

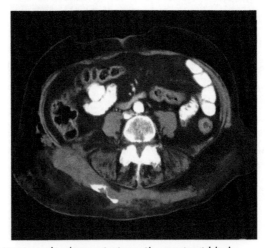

Fig. 8. Computed tomography demonstrates active contrast blush.

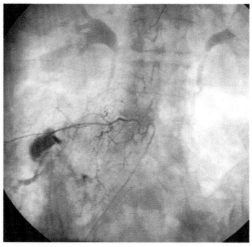

Fig. 9. Angiography demonstrating distal lumbar artery injury treated with coil embolization.

accomplished with a bed sheet or a commercially available binder. However, lateral compression pelvic fractures are usually not displaced. Therefore, there is little hemostatic advantage to placing the binder.

The astute clinician should have a high degree of suspicion for pelvic fracture hemorrhage in older patients who present with any signs of bleeding. There may be minimal findings on initial physical examination, because lateral compression pelvic fractures are often skeletally stable (**Figs. 7–9**). Thus, the pelvis will not move with initial physical examination. Transfusion therapy should be empiric and should occur early in patients with pelvic fracture hemorrhage. Because pelvic binders are of minimal help, institutional resources should be mobilized early to provide angiographic embolization for pelvic fracture hemorrhage. However, despite all efforts, elderly patients with pelvic fractures have a substantially higher mortality than do their younger counterparts.

REFERENCES

1. Robersten LZ. Falls in older people: epidemiology, risk factors and strategies for prevention. Age Ageing 2006;35(Suppl 2):ii37–41.
2. Aschkenasy MT, Rothenhaus TC. Trauma and falls in the elderly. Emerg Med Clin North Am 2006;24:413–32.
3. Gage BF, Birman-Deych E, Radford M, et al. Risk of osteoporotic failure in elderly patients taken warfarin. Arch Intern Med 2006;166:241–6.
4. Mears SC, Berry DJ. Outcomes of displaced and nondisplaced pelvic and sacral fractures in elderly adults. J Am Geriatr Soc 2011;59:1309–12.
5. Alexandru D, So W. Evaluation and management of vertebral compression fractures. Perm J 2012;16:46–51.
6. Johnell O, Kanis JA. An estimate of the worldwide problems, mortality and disabilities associated with hip fractures. Osteoporos Int 2014;15:897–902.
7. Nguyen TV, Center JR, Sambrook PN, et al. Risk factors for proximal humerus, forearm and wrist fractures in elderly men and women. The Dubbo Osteoporosis Epidemiology Study. Am J Epidemiol 2001;153:587–95.

8. Scalea TM, Simon HM, Duncan AO, et al. Geriatric blunt multiple trauma. Improved survival with early invasive monitoring. J Trauma 1990;30:129–36.

9. Rivers E, Nguyan B, Haystad S, et al. Early goal directed therapy in the treatment of severe sepsis and septic shock. N Engl J Med 2001;341:1368–77.

10. Havaldar R, Pilli SC, Putti BB. Effects of ageing on bone mineral composition and bone strength. IOSR J Dent Med Sci 2012;1:12–6.

11. Recker RR, Davies KM, Hinders SM. Bone gain in young adult women. JAMA 1992;268:2403–8.

12. O'Flaherty E. Modeling normal ageing bone loss with consideration of bone loss in osteoporosis. Toxicol Sci 2000;55:171–88.

13. Halbreich U, Palter S. Accelerated osteoporosis in psychiatric patients. Possible pathophysiological process. Schizophr Bull 1996;22:441–54.

14. Cummings SR, Nevitt MC, Brownser WS, et al. Risk factors for hip fractures in white women: study of osteoporosis Fracture Research Group. N Engl J Med 1995;332:767–73.

15. Guadalupe-Grau A, Fuentes T, Guerra B, et al. Exercise and bone mass in adults. Sports Med 2009;39:439–68.

16. Simon LS. Osteoporosis. Rheum Dis Clin North Am 2007;33:149–76.

17. Sweet MC, Sweet JM, Jeremiah MH, et al. Diagnosis and treatment of osteoporosis. Am Fam Physician 2009;79:193–200.

18. Seibel R, Laduca J, Hassett JM, et al. Blunt multiple trauma (ISS e6), femur traction and the pulmonary failure septic state. Ann Surg 1985;202:283–95.

19. Scalea TM, Scott JD, Brumback RJ, et al. Early fracture fixation may be "just fine" after head injury: No differences in CNS outcomes. J Trauma 1999;46:839–46.

20. Scalea TM, Boswell SA, Scott JD, et al. External fixation as a bridge to intramedullary nailing in poly-trauma patients with femur fractures. Damage control orthopedics. J Trauma 2000;48:613–23.

21. Scalea TM. Optimal timing of fracture fixation: have we learned anything in the past 20 years? J Trauma 2008;65:253–60.

22. Lefaivre KA, Macadam SA, Davidson DJ, et al. Length of stay, mortality, morbidity and delay to surgery in hip fractures. J Bone Joint Surg Br 2009;91:922–7.

23. Simunovic N, Devereaux PJ, Sprague S, et al. Effect of early surgery after hip fracture on mortality and complications: systematic review and meta-analysis. CMAJ 2010;182:1609–16.

24. Moja L, Piatti A, Pecoraro V, et al. Timing matters in hip fracture surgery: Patients operated within 48 hours have better outcomes. A meta-analysis and meta-regression of over 190,000 patients. PLoS One 2012;7:e46175. http://dx.doi.org/10.1371/journal.pone.0046175.

25. Leung F, Lau TW, Kwan K, et al. Does timing of surgery matter in fragility hip fractures? Osteoporos Int 2010;21:S529–34.

26. Henry SM, Pollak AN, Jones AL, et al. Pelvic fractures in geriatric patients: a distant clinical entity. J Trauma 2002;53:15–20.

Hematologic Issues in the Geriatric Surgical Patient

Philbert Y. Van, MD, Martin A. Schreiber, MD*

KEYWORDS

- Coagulopathy • Reversal of oral anticoagulants • Elderly

KEY POINTS

- Perform a thorough history and physical examination to uncover hematologic disorders.
- Nutritional deficiencies in elderly patients can lead to coagulopathy.
- Elderly patients with chronic disease, autoimmune disease, or malignancy are at risk for acquiring hematologic disorders.
- An increasing number of patients are prescribed oral anticoagulant/antiplatelet medications.
- There are no US Food and Drug Administration (FDA) approved reversal agents for the new oral anticoagulant medications, but known procoagulant agents with other FDA indications may be effective.

INTRODUCTION

The elderly population in the United States is expanding, with 43.1 million older than 65 years in 2012 expanding to an estimated 83.7 million by 2050. About 20% of the population will be older than 65 years in 2030.[1] This statistic translates to more elderly patients requiring surgical care and more elderly trauma patients. The elderly have acquired abnormalities in platelets and coagulation factor function as well as an increased incidence of systemic disease. Elderly patients are also more likely to take anticoagulant or antiplatelet medications.[2] Approximately 1.5% of the US population is prescribed warfarin; however, patients 65 years or older have the highest use of this medication. Elderly anticoagulated patients make up 25% of all trauma-related deaths and have the highest rate of traumatic brain injury.[3] Therefore, it is essential to be familiar with congenital and acquired coagulopathies and the mechanism of action of the new oral anticoagulation medications.

Disclosures: nothing to disclose.
Division of Trauma, Critical Care & Acute Care Surgery, Department of Surgery, Oregon Health & Science University, 3181 Southwest Sam Jackson Park Road, Mail Code L-611, Portland, OR 97239-3098, USA
* Corresponding author.
E-mail address: schreibm@ohsu.edu

Surg Clin N Am 95 (2015) 129–138
http://dx.doi.org/10.1016/j.suc.2014.09.012
0039-6109/15/$ – see front matter © 2015 Elsevier Inc. All rights reserved.

VASCULAR DISORDERS

The preoperative physical examination or trauma activation secondary examination may show evidence of an underlying disorder, including petechiae, purpura, or ecchymoses on extensor surfaces of the upper extremities or legs. These skin lesions are caused by increased transmural pressure, degeneration, and loss of dermal collagen, with resulting fragility of cutaneous small vessels. There may be no associated abnormality of platelet or the coagulation system with these skin lesions.[4]

Accumulation of monoclonal free light chain fragments occurs in amyloidosis. These deposits accumulate in the endothelium, resulting in loss of elasticity. The resultant vascular fragility can place the patient at increased risk for bleeding after trauma or surgical procedures.[5] Periorbital purpura is a common physical finding in patients with amyloidosis.[2]

Isolated elderly people can suffer from nutritional deficiencies. A vitamin C deficiency can lead to scurvy. Vitamin C is essential for collagen turnover, acting as a cofactor for the conversion of hydroxyproline to proline. Signs of scurvy include purpuric lesions on the legs and bleeding gums. This disorder can mimic vasculitis and bleeding disorders. Vitamin B_{12} and folic acid deficiency can lead to pancytopenia, including thrombocytopenia. Folic acid deficiency can occur within a month in hospitalized patients. Deficiency in vitamin B_{12} is unusual, because body stores can last 3 to 4 years before depletion. Underlying causes of vitamin B_{12} deficiency include malabsorption in the ileum, atrophic gastritis, partial or total gastrectomy, and pernicious anemia.[6]

COAGULATION FACTOR DISORDERS

Chronic liver disease can lead to decreased synthetic function and a reduction of all coagulation factors except for factor VIII, which is produced in liver sinusoidal cells and endothelial cells throughout the body. The severity of coagulation abnormalities is dependent on the degree of hepatic parenchymal damage and liver dysfunction.

In addition to vitamin C deficiency, elderly patients with a poor diet are at risk for vitamin K deficiency. Vitamin K is required for the γ carboxylation of coagulation factors II, VII, IX, and X, and proteins C and S. Malignancy, renal failure, and antibiotic therapy can interfere with vitamin K production by intestinal flora. Deficiency may result in a prolonged prothrombin time (PT) or increased international normalized ratio (INR).

Acquired Hemophilia

Late presentation of congenital bleeding disorders is a rare event. A detailed history should capture those with hemophilia A or B. Acquired hemophilia occurs with IgG1 and IgG4 autoantibodies to factor VIII. It is a rare condition, with 1 per million per year across all age groups, but it is more common in elderly patients, with an incidence of 7 per million per year older than 65 years.[2] This disorder is usually associated with autoimmune disorders, rheumatoid arthritis, systemic lupus erythematosus (SLE), and hematologic malignancies. Gastrointestinal bleeding, retropharyngeal and retroperitoneal hematomas, subcutaneous hematomas, cerebral hemorrhage, and urogenital tract bleeding are common, but the clinical manifestations can range from asymptomatic to life-threatening bleeding. Acquired hemophilia can be distinguished from congenital hemophilia, in which intra-articular and intramuscular hemorrhages are more common. Laboratory evaluation shows a prolonged activation of the partial thromboplastin time (aPTT). A Bethesda assay can quantify the inhibitor to factor

VIII. If the Bethesda titer is low (<5 units/mL), large doses of factor VIII concentrate can be used to overcome the inhibitor. In patients with severe hemorrhage and a high Bethesda titer (>5 units/mL), prothrombin concentrates or recombinant factor VIIa (rfVIIa) may be needed.[7] The use of immunosuppression with steroids or cyclophosphamide is controversial. Immune suppression in the elderly population is not without risk, because of infectious morbidity and mortality.

Acquired von Willebrand Disease

Elderly patients with lymphoproliferative disorders, monoclonal gammopathies, and myeloproliferative disorders may develop an acquired von Willebrand disease. This is a rare condition, which is associated with postoperative or spontaneous hemorrhage, presenting with mucocutaneous and skin bleeding.[8,9] The pathophysiology is not well understood but involves autoantibodies directed against von Willebrand factor (vWF). Standard coagulation tests (PT, aPTT) are normal, but vWF ristocetin cofactor and vWF antigen are decreased. This rare disorder is treated with administration of desmopressin (DDAVP) and treatment of the underlying disease. Long-term treatment may require high-dose intravenous immunoglobulin (IVIG).

PLATELET DISORDERS

Because of an increased rate of destruction, decreased rate of production, and abnormal distribution of platelets, thrombocytopenia is one of the most common hemostatic abnormalities in elderly patients. The severity of hemorrhage is influenced by the degree of thrombocytopenia and the nature of qualitative deficits in platelet function. Pseudothrombocytopenia can occur when platelets clump together after being exposed to ethylenediaminetetraacetic acid used in vacuum tubes used for blood collection for complete blood counts.

Immune Thrombocytopenia Purpura

Circulating antiplatelet autoantibodies are responsible for the decreased platelet count. Platelets with the bound autoantibodies are then prematurely destroyed in the peripheral reticuloendothelial system. Immune thrombocytopenia purpura (ITP) is associated with lymphoproliferative disorders and autoimmune diseases. The adult form of ITP is different from the acute form of ITP in children, because there is no preceding systemic or viral illness. In the age group older than 60 to 74 years, the incidence of ITP is 2 per 100,000 per year.[2] This disease occurs in patients with SLE and chromic lymphocytic leukemia. Treatment is recommended only if the patient is symptomatic and the platelet count is less than 30,000. Administration of steroids and IVIG is the first-line therapy for ITP. Second-line treatment includes azathioprine, danazol, and dapsone. If medical management fails, a splenectomy may be indicated.

Posttransfusion Purpura

Posttransfusion purpura (PTP) is a rare complication of transfusion, resulting in severe thrombocytopenia 2 to 14 days after transfusion. Antihuman platelet antigen (anti-HPA) antibodies in the recipient are directed against donor platelets from the transfusion. These anti-HPA antibodies then cross-react with and destroy the recipient's platelets. Most patients are multiparous women.[6] PTP is diagnosed by testing for the presence of anti-HPA antibodies. This condition can be treated with IVIG and steroids. With the introduction of leukodepleted blood products, the incidence of PTP has decreased dramatically.

Thrombotic Thrombocytopenia Purpura

Fluctuating neurologic symptoms, renal insufficiency, fever, microangiopathic hemolytic anemia, and thrombocytopenia can all be present in thrombotic thrombocytopenia purpura (TTP). A relatively rare disorder with an incidence of 11.29 per million per year, this disorder is managed with plasma exchange.[10] Platelet transfusion is contraindicated, because it makes the syndrome worse. There are no diagnostic tests, but characteristic schistocytes on peripheral blood smears and increased lactate dehydrogenase levels are clues to this condition.

Myeloproliferative Disorders

These disorders include myelofibrosis, essential thrombocythemia, and polycythemia vera. Despite having a normal to increased platelet count, abnormal bleeding can occur in these patients.[11] Abnormal bleeding mainly involves the mucous membranes and skin. The incidence of bleeding complications in these disorders ranges from 1.7% to 37%. The thrombocytosis may cause an acquired von Willebrand syndrome, which may be the underlying cause of abnormal bleeding. Bleeding risks increase when the primary myeloproliferative disorder is poorly controlled.

Myelodysplastic Syndrome

This group of disorders primarily affects elderly patients. Ineffective hematopoiesis and peripheral cytopenias are the main characteristics of this syndrome. Because of both qualitative and quantitative platelet defects, patients are thrombocytopenic and have abnormal bleeding. Before surgical procedures, patients may benefit from platelet transfusion.[12]

Uremia

Impaired platelet function and platelet to vessel wall interaction can occur in uremia. Uremic toxins contribute to platelet dysfunction and can be improved with hemodialysis. Secondary treatments include administration of DDAVP, estrogens, cryoprecipitate, and platelet transfusions.

MEDICATION-INDUCED COAGULOPATHY

In the last several decades, the indications for anticoagulation and antiplatelet therapy have expanded. Although the coumarin derivatives and heparinoids are reversible, the newer anticoagulants and antiplatelet agents that have been approved for new indications have no specific mechanisms to reverse their effects. It is also important to inquire about herbal remedies during the history and physical examination. Garlic inhibits platelet aggregation and can increase fibrinolysis. Gingko inhibits platelet aggregation. Both garlic and gingko can increase bleeding when combined with other antiplatelet medications. Ginseng has been shown to reduce the anticoagulant effect of warfarin. St John's wort induces cytochrome P450, which can interfere with the metabolism of warfarin.[13]

With a larger number of anticoagulated patients and an expanded elderly population, more of the population is at risk for bleeding after trauma. It is important to be familiar with anticoagulants and antiplatelet agents and reversal protocols.

Warfarin (Coumadin)

This oral anticoagulant inhibits the vitamin K–dependent clotting factors II, VII, IX, and X, and proteins C and S. The INR measures the level of anticoagulation. It is used for prophylaxis and treatment of deep venous thrombosis (DVT), pulmonary embolus

(PE), thromboembolic complications associated with atrial fibrillation, and cardiac valve replacement. Warfarin is rapidly absorbed via the gastrointestinal tract and reaches maximum levels at 90 minutes. However, the dose-response relationship can be affected by diet, drug interactions, genetics, and environmental factors. Those patients on warfarin before traumatic injury have a higher mortality.[14] Transfusion of fresh frozen plasma (FFP) or prothrombin complex concentrate (PCC) is used for rapid reversal of warfarin.[15] PCC has several advantages over FFP: it is virally inactivated, it does not require thawing or blood typing, and it can achieve therapeutic levels with a smaller volume of infused medication.[16] Recently, the 4-factor PCC (Kcentra) has been approved by the US Food and Drug Administration (FDA) for urgent reversal of warfarin. Vitamin K can also be used to accelerate production of the dependent clotting factors. The recommendation for patients undergoing elective surgery is to stop warfarin 5 days before scheduled surgery and bridge with enoxaparin if indicated.

Unfractionated Heparin

Heparin binds antithrombin III (ATIII) to form a complex that inactivates factors IIa, IXa, Xa, XIa, and XIIa. Because of plasma protein binding and nonuniform fraction size, heparin has a variable response and must be monitored with serial aPTT measurements. Heparin therapy is indicated for prophylaxis and treatment of DVT and PE, treatment of atrial fibrillation with embolization, prophylaxis against clotting during cardiac and vascular surgery, and the prophylaxis and treatment of peripheral arterial embolism. The only FDA-approved antidote is protamine sulfate. FFP should not be used for reversal of heparin anticoagulation, because it contains antithrombin, which may potentiate hemorrhage.

Enoxaparin (Lovenox), Low-Molecular-Weight Heparin

Low-molecular-weight heparins (LMWH) have a slightly different mechanism of action compared with unfractionated heparin. Enoxaparin binds to ATIII, but because of its smaller molecular size, it is not as effective as unfractionated heparin in inhibiting thrombin. However, LMWH has higher anti–factor Xa activity. When given subcutaneously, enoxaparin has 90% bioavailability and has a half-life of 3 to 6 hours. Prophylaxis with LMWH has the same indications as heparin. LMWH has gained popularity in use over unfractionated heparin, because enoxaparin does not require routine monitoring. Measurement of anti–factor Xa levels is recommended for obesity, renal failure, and pregnancy, although recent data suggest that anti-Xa levels may not correlate with drug efficacy.[17] LMWH is FDA approved for DVT prophylaxis in abdominal surgery, hip and knee arthroplasty, inpatient and outpatient treatment of DVT with or without PE, prophylaxis of ischemic complications of unstable angina and non-Q wave myocardial infarction, and treatment of acute ST-segment elevation myocardial infarction. Enoxaparin is metabolized by the liver and cleared via the kidneys. There is no FDA-approved antidote for enoxaparin. Protamine sulfate is successful in partial reversal, and rFVIIa has been reported to be effective as well.[18]

Aspirin

Aspirin irreversibly inactivates cyclooxygenase 1 (COX-1) on platelets. Inhibition of COX-1 prevents the synthesis of thromboxane A_2, which is a platelet aggregator and vasoconstrictor. The medication is metabolized rapidly, but effects last until there are at least 20% new platelets in circulation.[19] Aspirin therapy is indicated for cerebrovascular and cardiovascular disease, autoimmune and rheumatologic disorders, and

Table 1
Anticoagulant/antiplatelet reversal agents

Reversal Agent	Mechanism of Action	Availability	Time to Onset	Adverse Effects	Uses	Disadvantages
Vitamin K (Mephyton)	Required for synthesis of factors II, VII, IX, X	Readily	2–24 h	Anaphylaxis, hypotension, skin reactions	Reversal of warfarin	Slow onset of effect
Protamine	Binds to heparin	Readily	Minutes	Bradycardia, hypotension, anaphylaxis, leukopenia, thrombocytopenia	Reversal of heparin, partial reversal of LMWH[a]	Short half-life of medication, slow administration
FFP	Provides vitamin K-dependent clotting factors	Readily, but requires blood typing and thawing	Minutes	Congestive heart failure, transfusion related acute lung injury, ABO mismatch	Reversal of warfarin	Long preparation time, large volumes required
Platelets	Replenish platelets in circulation	Limited in small or rural institutions	Unknown	ABO mismatch, infection, alloimmunization,	Restore platelet function after aspirin or clopidogrel use[a]	Insufficient evidence for improved outcome
rfVIIa (Novoseven)	Binds to platelets, increases thrombin generation	Limited	Minutes	Thrombosis, anaphylaxis, hypotension, fever, injection site reaction	Reversal of heparin, warfarin, fondaparinux, dabigatran[a]	Expensive, optimal dose not established

	Composition/mechanism	Availability	Time to effect	Adverse effects	Indication	Limitations
4-factor PCC (Kcentra)	Factor II, VII, IX, and X, proteins C and S	May be limited in some institutions	Minutes	Thromboembolism, hypotension, anemia, nausea, emesis, headache, tachycardia, bronchospasm	Reversal of warfarin	Limited availability
PCC (Profilnine)	Factor II, IX, X; small amounts of factor VII	May be limited in some institutions	Minutes	Injection site reaction, fever, anaphylaxis, angioedema, thromboembolism, nephrotic syndrome	Reversal of warfarin,[a] rivaroxaban, dabigatran	Optimal dosing not established, limited availability
FEIBA	Nonactivated factors II, IX, X; activated factor VII: enhances thrombin generation	Limited	Minutes	Anaphylaxis, hypersensitivity, thromboembolism,	Reversal of rivaroxaban,[a] dabigatran	No established monitoring test, metabolism and excretion unknown

[a] Off-label use of medication.

Data from Gordon JL, Fabian TC, Lee MD, et al. Anticoagulant and antiplatelet medications encountered in emergency surgery patients: a review of reversal strategies. J Trauma Acute Care Surg 2013;75(3):475–86.

postrevascularization procedures (carotid endarterectomy, coronary artery bypass grafting, and percutaneous angioplasty). There is no FDA-approved antidote, but some intracranial hemorrhage data advocate platelet transfusion to reverse the effects of aspirin by providing platelets with COX-1 activity.[15,20]

Clopidogrel (Plavix)

This medication is activated by the liver and subsequently blocks the binding of adenosine diphosphate (ADP) to platelets and its release from platelets. Without the release of ADP, platelets cannot be activated. The half-life of clopidogrel is 6.5 hours, but the antiplatelet effect can last up to 5 days. Clopidogrel is FDA approved for unstable angina and non-ST-segment elevation myocardial infarction, ST-segment elevation myocardial infarction, and patients with a recent history of myocardial infarction, recent stroke, or peripheral arterial disease. Clopidogrel is also used in conjunction with aspirin to prevent restenosis of coronary artery stents. Current recommendations are for 6 months of combined aspirin and clopidogrel therapy for bare metal stents and 1 year for drug-eluting stents. Clopidogrel should be stopped 7 days before elective surgery. Because of its irreversible blockade of ADP binding and release, there is no antidote for clopidogrel. Because preinjury clopidogrel use is associated with significantly higher mortality in elderly patients with trauma, transfusion of platelets is advocated.[15,21]

Fondaparinux (Arixtra), Indirect Factor Xa Inhibitor

This medication is administered subcutaneously and binds to antithrombin to inactivate factor Xa and then in turn inhibits thrombin formation. Fondaparinux has greater anti–factor Xa activity than enoxaparin. Onset of action is within 30 minutes and the half-life ranges from 17 to 21 hours, which allows for once-a-day dosing. The duration of effect is approximately 48 hours. Fondaparinux-specific anti–factor Xa assays are available, but no therapeutic anti-Xa range has been established. There is no cross-reaction with heparin-induced thrombocytopenia (HIT) antibodies; therefore, fondaparinux can be used in patients with HIT needing anticoagulation. Fondaparinux is FDA approved for DVT prophylaxis in abdominal surgery, hip and knee arthroplasty, hip fracture repair, and treatment of DVT or acute PE until a therapeutic INR is reached on warfarin. No FDA-approved antidote exists for fondaparinux, but an in vitro study showed full reversal with factor eight inhibitor bypassing activity (FEIBA) and no effect with PCC.[22] Several case studies have reported successful reversal with rFVIIa.[15,23,24]

Rivaroxaban (Xarelto) and Apixaban (Eliquis), Direct Factor Xa Inhibitors

These oral medications exert their anticoagulation effect by directly binding factor Xa, inhibiting its activity without needing antithrombin as a cofactor. The half-life ranges from 9 to 19 hours, and the medication is metabolized by the liver and excreted via urine and feces. There is no routine monitoring assay for this class of medication. Rivaroxaban and apixaban are FDA approved for use in reducing risk of stroke and systemic embolism in patients with atrial fibrillation. Rivaroxaban is also used for DVT prophylaxis in surgical patients. There are no FDA-approved antidotes for either rivaroxaban or apixaban. PCC has been used successfully in a few patients on rivaroxaban.[25] For apixaban, there are limited data on use of FFP, rFVIIa, and PCC for reversal of anticoagulation.[26]

Dabigatran (Pradaxa), Direct Thrombin Inhibitor

Dabigatran is an oral anticoagulant that inhibits free and clot-bound thrombin as well as thrombin-induced platelet aggregation. Because dabigatran is not bound to plasma proteins, it has a more predictable response compared with heparinoids. It is excreted via the kidneys and has a half-life of 12 to 17 hours, assuming normal renal function. This medication is FDA approved for prevention of recurrent DVT and prophylaxis for stroke and systemic embolism in patients with atrial fibrillation. No routine monitoring of dabigatran is recommended. There is no FDA-approved antidote for direct thrombin inhibitors.[27] A few studies have shown success in reversal of dabigatran with FEIBA, PCC, and rFVIIa (**Table 1**).[22,28]

SUMMARY

The population of Americans older than 65 years in 2012 is projected to increase by 200% to more than 80 million by the year 2050. Geriatric patients are at risk for bleeding complications both after surgery and traumatic injuries because of acquired coagulation disorders and use of anticoagulation and antiplatelet medications. Chronic systemic diseases, malignancy, nutritional deficiency, and autoimmune diseases can result in coagulation factor deficiencies, vascular disorders, platelet dysfunction, and acquired hemophilia in the elderly population. The surgeon must not overlook these potential coagulation and platelet disorders when scheduling elderly patients for elective or urgent procedures, or evaluating an elderly patient with trauma. With expanding indications for the use of oral anticoagulants and antiplatelet medications, increasing numbers of geriatric patients are at risk for hemorrhagic complications after traumatic injury. It is essential that surgeons are familiar with the new classes of anticoagulants and their mechanism of action: factor Xa inhibitors and direct thrombin inhibitors. Although there are no FDA-approved reversal agents for clopidogrel, rivaroxaban, apixaban, dabigatran, and enoxaparin, clinicians must continue to keep up to date with the off-label uses of PCC, 4-factor PCC, platelets, FEIBA, and rFVIIa as antidotes for these medications.

REFERENCES

1. US Census Bureau. Fueled by aging baby boomers, nation's older population to nearly double, census bureau reports. Available at: http://www.census.gov/newsroom/releases/archives/aging_population/cb14-84.html. Accessed May 30, 2014.
2. Nicolle AL, Talks KL, Hanley JP. Congenital and acquired bleeding problems in elderly patients. Reviews in Clinical Gerontology 2005;15:9–26.
3. Fortuna GR, Mueller EW, James LE, et al. The impact of preinjury antiplatelet and anticoagulant pharmacotherapy on outcomes in elderly patients with hemorrhagic brain injury. Surgery 2008;144:598–605.
4. Hussain S. Disorders of hemostasis and thrombosis in the aged. Med Clin North Am 1976;60:1273–87.
5. Mumford AD, ODonnell J, Gillmore JD, et al. Bleeding symptoms and coagulation abnormalities in 337 patients with AL amyloidosis. Br J Haematol 2000;100:454–60.
6. Anderson JA, Lee AY. Hemorrhagic disorders. In: Halter JB, editor. Hazzard's geriatric medicine and gerontology. 6th edition. New York: McGraw-Hill; 2009. p. 1253–66.
7. Franchini M. Acquired hemophilia A. Hematology 2006;11(2):119–25.
8. Kumar S, Pruthi RK, Nichols WL. Acquired von Willebrand disease. Mayo Clin Proc 2002;77:181–7.
9. Lison S, Dietrich W, Spannagl M. Unexpected bleeding in the operating room: the role of acquired von Willebrand disease. Anesth Analg 2012;114(1):73–81.

10. Terrell DR, Williams LA, Vesely SK, et al. The incidence of thrombotic thrombocytopenic purpura-hemolytic uremic syndrome: all patients, idiopathic patients, and patients with severe ADAMTS-13 deficiency. J Thromb Haemost 2005;3:1432–6.

11. Elliot MA, Tefferi A. Thrombosis and haemorrhage in polycythemia vera and essential thrombocythaemia. Br J Haematol 2005;128:275–90.

12. Bowen D, Culligan D, Jowitt S. Guidelines for the diagnosis and therapy of adult myelodysplastic syndromes. Br J Haematol 2003;120:187–200.

13. Ang-Lee MK, Moss J, Chun-Su Y. Herbal medicines and perioperative care. JAMA 2001;286(2):208–16.

14. Dossett LA, Riesel JN, Griffin MR, et al. Prevalence and implications of preinjury warfarin use: an analysis of the National Trauma Databank. Arch Surg 2011; 146(5):565–70.

15. Beshay JE, Morgan H, Madden C, et al. Emergency reversal of anticoagulation and antiplatelet therapies in neurosurgical patients: a review. J Neurosurg 2010;112:307–18.

16. Sarode R, Milling TJ, Rafaai MA, et al. Efficacy and safety of a 4-factor prothrombin complex concentrate in patients on vitamin K antagonists presenting with major bleeding: a randomized, plasma-controlled, phase IIIb study. Circulation 2013;128:1234–43.

17. Van PY, Cho SD, Underwood SJ, et al. Thrombelastography versus anti-factor Xa levels in the assessment of prophylactic-dose enoxaparin in critically ill patients. J Trauma 2009;66(6):1509–17.

18. Gordon JL, Fabian TC, Lee MD, et al. Anticoagulant and antiplatelet medications encountered in emergency surgery patients: a review of reversal strategies. J Trauma Acute Care Surg 2013;75(3):475–86.

19. McMillian WD, Rogers FB. Management of prehospital antiplatelet and anticoagulant therapy in traumatic head injury: a review. J Trauma 2009;66:942–50.

20. Campbell PG, Sen A, Yadla S, et al. Emergency reversal of antiplatelet agents in patients presenting with an intracranial hemorrhage: a clinical review. World Neurosurg 2010;74(2-3):279–85.

21. Wong DK, Lurie F, Wong LL. The effects of clopidogrel on elderly traumatic brain injured patients. J Trauma 2008;65:1303–8.

22. Mancl EE, Crawford AN, Voils SA. Contemporary anticoagulation reversal: focus on direct thrombin inhibitors and factor Xa inhibitors. J Pharm Pract 2012;26: 43–51.

23. Harder S, Klinkhardt U, Alvarez JM. Avoidance of bleeding during surgery in patients receiving anticoagulant and/or antiplatelet therapy: pharmacokinetic and pharmacodynamics considerations. Clin Pharmacokinet 2004;43(14):963–81.

24. Bijsterveld NR, Moons AH, Boekholdt SM, et al. Ability of recombinant factor VIIa to reverse the anticoagulant effect of the pentasaccharide fondaparinux in healthy volunteers. Circulation 2002;106(20):2550–4.

25. Eerenberg ES, Kamphuisen PW, Sijpkens MK, et al. Reversal of rivaroxaban and dabigatran by prothrombin complex concentrate. Circulation 2011;124:1573–9.

26. Kaatz S, Kouides PA, Garcia DA, et al. Guidance on the emergent reversal of oral thrombin and factor Xa inhibitors. Am J Hematol 2012;87(S1):S141–5.

27. Hankey GJ, Eikelboom JW. Dabigatran etexilate: a new oral thrombin inhibitor. Circulation 2011;123:1436–50.

28. Khoo TL, Weatherburn C, Kershaw G, et al. The use of FEIBA in the correction of coagulation abnormalities induced by dabigatran. Int J Lab Hematol 2013;35(2): 222–4.

Pharmacology for the Geriatric Surgical Patient

Janine Then, PharmD[a], Samuel A. Tisherman, MD[b],*

KEYWORDS

- Geriatrics • Surgery • Pharmacology • Adverse drug reactions

KEY POINTS

- Physical changes with age alter how medications act and are metabolized by the body.
- The elderly are at increased risk of experiencing an adverse effect of medications, especially during the postoperative period when additional medications are added to their regimen.
- All medications used in the elderly should be dose adjusted to account for altered pharmacokinetics and should be titrated to the lowest effective dose for the shortest appropriate duration.

INTRODUCTION

The elderly make up a significant proportion of the population in the United States. In 2011, adults older than 65 years made up 13.3% of the United States population or approximately 41.1 million, and those over the age of 85 comprised about 5.7 million people. The elderly are also living healthier lives, with 44% of noninstitutionalized elderly describing their health as very good or excellent (http://www.aoa.gov/Aging_Statistics/. Accessed 3/13/2014.)

Unfortunately, the elderly are at increased risk of experiencing an adverse drug reaction (ADR). ADRs may account for up to 24% of hospitalizations in the elderly. Approximately 1 in 6 elderly patients will experience an ADR during admission to hospital.[1,2] ADRs in the elderly often present in an atypical manner and are nonspecific. A single ADR can increase a patient's length of stay in hospital by an average of 6.2 days.[3]

Many ADRs are preventable, as they are based on the known mechanism of action and/or predictable decreased clearance of the medication, withdrawal of a chronic

a Department of Pharmacy and Therapeutics, University of Pittsburgh, 3501 Terrace St, Pittsburgh, PA 15261, USA; b Department of Surgery, University of Maryland, 22 S. Greene St, Baltimore, MD 21201, USA
* Corresponding author.
E-mail address: stisherman@umm.edu

Surg Clin N Am 95 (2015) 139–147
http://dx.doi.org/10.1016/j.suc.2014.09.013
0039-6109/15/$ – see front matter © 2015 Elsevier Inc. All rights reserved.
surgical.theclinics.com

medication, or a drug-drug interaction.[1] Awareness of common physiologic changes and common drug-drug interactions seen in the elderly may help prevent ADRs in geriatric surgical patients (**Box 1**).

CHANGES IN PHARMACOKINETICS AND PHARMACODYNAMICS

Aging is not a single process, so as individuals age their interindividual variability accumulates. This variation creates differences in response to physiologic stress. The ease with which elderly patients tolerate surgery is related to their specific aging process. In general, the elderly experience many physiologic changes that affect their ability to metabolize and use medications (**Tables 1** and **2**). The frail elderly require even more caution when dosing and using medications.

Absorption and Bioavailability

Saliva production and gastric acid secretion are thought to be reduced as a result of aging. Although this theoretically could cause less drug to be available for absorption because of changes in ionization, in clinical practice this change seems to have little effect on medications used in the geriatric patient. Alternatively, these changes may be more frequent in frail patients and do not apply to healthy older patients who lack comorbid conditions.[4]

Oral bioavailability is not only determined by the amount of drug present in the gastrointestinal (GI) tract but also whether the absorbed drug undergoes first-pass hepatic metabolism before systemic distribution. First-pass metabolism reduces the amount of drug reaching the systemic circulation, thus reducing bioavailability. This first-pass metabolism may be impaired by decreased blood flow to the liver or by decreased activity of hepatic enzymes, leading to a decreased amount of drug extracted.[5] In turn this may lead to higher serum concentrations of certain medications (eg, propranolol and labetalol).[4]

Distribution

Body composition changes over time. As the body ages, total body fat increases at the expense of lean body mass and total body water. These changes lead to a smaller volume of distribution and, consequently, higher drug concentration for hydrophilic medications such as digoxin, but larger volumes of distribution for lipophilic medications such as lidocaine, phenytoin, and benzodiazepines.[1,4,5] The distribution of these medications into the adipose tissue may lead to a delayed effect of the medication.

Box 1
Common drug classes associated with adverse drug reactions

- Antibiotics
- Digoxin
- Antihyperglycemic agents
- Anticoagulants/Antithrombotics
- Diuretics
- Nonsteroidal anti-inflammatory agents

Adapted from Petrovic M, van der Camme T, Onder G. Adverse drug reactions in older people: detection and prevention. Drugs Aging 2012;29:454.

Table 1
Age-related changes that affect pharmacokinetics

Change in Elderly Patients Compared with Younger Patients	Possible Effect of Changes on Drug Concentration in the Elderly
Decreased gastric acid production	Increase or decrease depending on medication
Decreased gastric blood flow	Decreased adsorption
Decreased first-pass effect	Increased availability of active drugs; decreased availability of drugs requiring activation
Increased body fat	Decrease lipophilic medications
Decreased lean body mass/total body water	Increase hydrophilic medications
Decreased albumin	Increase unbound (active) drug
Decreased size of liver and blood flow	Increase
Glomerular filtration rate	Increase
Tubular function	Decrease

However, after the medication is discontinued it may be slowly released from the adipose stores, leading to prolonged therapeutic effects.[6]

Changes in the serum proteins, albumin and α1-acid glycoprotein, can also alter the amount of active drug in the body. The effect of alterations in protein binding is generally only observed in the frail elderly and may be more related to disease states than the aging process per se, because renal disease, liver disease, and even diabetes mellitus are known to alter drug binding. In these patients, however, toxicity may be observed for medications such as phenytoin, digoxin, and warfarin despite total drug levels being in the therapeutic range.[6] Monitoring free (nonprotein bound) drug levels should be considered in the frail elderly when possible.

Besides the chemical properties of a medication, transporter proteins such as P-glycoprotein are integral to the ability of a drug to cross the blood-brain barrier and other tissues. P-glycoprotein, like many other enzymes, seems to have decreased activity with aging. At present, however, there is no known clinical consequence of this potential decrease in activity.[5]

Table 2
Examples of pharmacodynamics changes in the elderly

Medication	Pharmacodynamic Effect	Change in Elderly
Diazepam	Sedation, postural sway	Increased
Diltiazem	Antihypertensive effects	Increased
Diphenhydramine	Postural sway	Increased
Furosemide	Diuretic response	Decreased
Heparin	Anticoagulation effects	No change
Isoproterenol	Chronotropic effects	Decreased
Phenylephrine	α-Adrenergic response	No change
Temazepam	Postural sway	Increased
Verapamil	Antihypertensive effects	Increased
Warfarin	Anticoagulant effects	Increased

Metabolism

There are clear changes in various organs as they age. The liver decreases in size as well as hepatic blood flow. This reduction in perfusion can slow the rate at which medications are delivered to the liver for metabolism. Declines in the function of the various cytochrome P450 isoenzymes that account for phase I metabolism appear in both the frail and healthy elderly. Studies to characterize the percentage decline in individual isozymes are limited by genetic differences in patients who appear to physiologically age at different rates, and other factors such as smoking status, ethnicity, and sex.[4,5] Unfortunately, at this time there are no routine clinical tests that can aid in determining the amount of liver impairment in a specific patient.

In healthy patients through 80 years of age there appears to be little decline in phase II metabolism, which is responsible for glucuronidation, acetylation, and sulfation.[4] Esterases found throughout the body in various tissues and in the plasma do not show a decline in function in healthy elderly patients, but are significantly reduced in the frail elderly and those patients having suffered hip fractures, delirium, and even pneumonia.[6]

Elimination

Aging is associated with a reduction in the number of renal glomeruli (see article by Baldea AJ, elsewhere in this issue). Despite this reduction in number, about one-third of elderly patients will maintain their glomerular filtration rate (GFR) through almost 90 years of age. In a small percentage of patients, GFR increases with age.[5,6] Declines in GFR seem to be most related to concomitant diseases, such as hypertension, chronic heart failure, and diabetes mellitus.[5] Although frailty may be related to decreasing GFR, it is as yet unknown whether it is a consequence or a cause of renal impairment.[6]

Tubular secretion and reabsorption may decrease in the elderly, although these parameters are not well characterized or assessed by current methods of estimating GFR. Decreases in renal function may also lead to alterations in liver metabolism of certain medications, as a result of either reduced gene expression or shifting of clearance from the renal system to the hepatic system.[4]

Pharmacodynamics

A drug's action in the body can be affected by the aging process. For example, the elderly have a decreased response to verapamil's effects on cardiac conduction but an increased response to its vasodilator properties. β-Adrenoceptor responsiveness is also decreased in the elderly, and seems to be related to reductions in cyclic adenosine monophosphate after receptor stimulation. α-Adrenoceptors do not appear to be affected by aging.[4]

Despite similar plasma concentration in young and elderly patients, there is greater inhibition of clotting factors in the presence of warfarin and increased sedation in the presence of diazepam.[4,6] The mechanisms for these effects are unknown at present.

PREOPERATIVE ISSUES

A complete medication history is imperative before elective surgery. The elderly take on average 2 to 5 prescription medications daily.[5] Those who are institutionalized may take closer to 7 pharmacologic agents daily. Unfortunately, this does not account for all medications that an elderly patient may be using regularly. The elderly use 3 times more over-the-counter preparations and twice the number of alternative/herbal preparations in comparison with the population in general.[2]

Medication allergies and previous ADRs should also be investigated before surgery to prevent similar drugs from being prescribed during the perioperative period. Reactions to medications should be discussed and documented to distinguish between true allergies and intolerances.

A plan should be created to address long-term medications that cannot or should not be stopped abruptly if the likelihood is that the patient will not be able to resume oral medications immediately postoperatively. Specific examples include β-blockers, antidepressants, antipsychotics, and anxiolytics. The elderly may be at increased risk of postoperative atrial fibrillation caused by age and comorbidities. The abrupt discontinuation of β-blockers can further increase the risk of postoperative atrial fibrillation.[7]

For patients on anticoagulant or antiplatelet therapy, the associated bleeding risk of the surgery should be weighed against the risk of discontinuing the agent, which is predicated on the indication for the agent. Ideally a plan should be devised jointly by the surgeon and the prescribing physician to determine the length of time to hold long-term therapy and to determine whether bridging therapy is appropriate (**Table 3**).

POSTOPERATIVE ISSUES

The risk of ADRs is greatest after an elderly patient's operation, owing to the introduction of new medications, including anesthetics, analgesics, antiemetics, and chemoprophylaxis for deep venous thrombosis. In addition, fluid resuscitation can significantly increase the volume of distribution of medications, leading to underdosing. On the other hand, postoperative renal or hepatic dysfunction can decrease metabolism, leading to toxicity.

Medications added to treat postoperative complications, such as atrial fibrillation, delirium, or infections, can further increase risk. When a patient is taking only 2 medications concurrently, the estimated risk of an ADR is 13%, but this risk increases to

Table 3
Potential management of newer anticoagulants before surgery

Drug	Renal Function	Low Bleeding Risk Surgery	High Bleeding Risk Surgery
Dabigatran 150 mg BID	Normal to mild impairment (CrCl >50 mL/min)	Skip 2 doses	Skip 4 doses
Dabigatran 150 mg BID	Moderate impairment (CrCl 30–50 mL/min)	Skip 4 doses	Skip 6–8 doses
Rivaroxaban 20 mg QD	Normal to mild impairment (>50 mL/min)	Skip 1 dose	Skip 2 doses
Rivaroxaban 15 mg QD	Moderate impairment (30–50 mL/min)	Skip 1 dose	Skip 2 doses
Rivaroxaban 15 mg QD	Severe impairment (CrCl 15–29 mL/min)	Skip 2 doses	Skip 3 doses
Apixaban 5 mg BID	Normal or mild impairment (>50 mL/min)	Skip 2 doses	Skip 4 doses
Apixaban 5 mg BID	Moderate impairment (30–50 mL/min)	Skip 4 doses	Skip 6 doses

Abbreviations: BID, twice daily; CrCl, creatinine clearance; QD, every day.
Adapted from Spyropoulos AC, Douketis JD. How I treat anticoagulated patients undergoing an elective procedure or surgery. Blood 2012;120:2959.

82% with 7 medications.[1] Each medication added may have its own adverse effects and/or may interact with a medication that the patient is already receiving.

In the elderly it is important to not overtreat. The worst scenario occurs when additional medications are used to treat adverse reactions from other medications, leading to an iatrogenic cascade. It is crucial to investigate why the patient has a new symptom.[2]

Pain

Pain is subjective and completely known only to the patient experiencing it. Pain assessment in the elderly is complicated by cognitive impairment, communication difficulties, and cultural differences. Pain-intensity scales can be used in most patients without severe cognitive impairment, but may require more patience and time to complete with the elderly patient. Physical cues that a patient is in pain may be present, but if a patient has a chronic pain syndrome, common clinical signs such as tachycardia and hypertension may be absent.[8] For patients who are impaired, family input can be helpful in some circumstances.

Multimodal therapy may be especially important in the elderly (**Table 4**). A combination of weaker and stronger analgesics along with adjuvant and nonpharmacologic treatments may decrease the risk of severe adverse reactions.[8]

Delirium is frequently considered an adverse effect of opioid medications. In some studies, the risk of delirium was increased in patients receiving opioids in comparison with those who did not. By contrast, other studies have suggested that underdosing of opiates increased the risk of delirium. Patients with severe pain appear to have a significantly increased risk of delirium. Adequate treatment of pain and appropriate selection of medication are critical for decreasing the risk of delirium in the elderly.[9]

Table 4
Precautions for the elderly taking pain medications

Drug	Precaution	Recommendation
Acetaminophen	Metabolism maintained in healthy elderly; caution in frail, malnourished, dehydrated, and high alcohol consumption	May benefit most from scheduled doses; maintain strict 4 g limit in 24 h; consider lower doses (2–3 g max/24 h) in high-risk groups
NSAIDs	Elderly seem to be at higher risk of GI bleeding, renal dysfunction, and prolonged half-lives of some agents	Short half-life agents such as ibuprofen or diclofenac, given at the lowest effective dose for a short duration, may decrease risk but close monitoring required
Tramadol	Associated with delirium, seizures, dizziness, nausea/vomiting Requires renal dose adjustment and activation by the liver to its active form	May have fewer respiratory and GI adverse effects but dose adjustments required in renal dysfunction
Opioids	Most opioids are metabolized in the liver and excreted renally Increased risk of falls with injury when opioids are initiated	Use of short-acting agents that can quickly be titrated to adequate pain control may decrease delirium

Abbreviations: GI, gastrointestinal; NSAIDs, nonsteroidal anti-inflammatory drugs.

The ideal pain medication in the elderly would have a predictable half-life, no active metabolites, and be easily titratable. Agents such as morphine and meperidine have active metabolites and should be used sparingly in elderly patients, especially those with renal impairment. Oxycodone, hydromorphone, and fentanyl are generally recommended, even in patients with impaired renal function.[8,9]

Tapentadol, meperidine, tramadol, fentanyl, and oxycodone have the potential to interact with serotonin reuptake inhibitors, and potentially lead to serotonin syndrome.[10] Codeine and tramadol require activation by the liver, which may be impaired because of drug interactions or frailty.[9]

The elderly should also be monitored for constipation, nausea, and dizziness while receiving pain medications. A bowel regimen should include a stimulant or osmotic laxative, such as senna or polyethylene glycol, and should be started as soon as possible after initiation of opioid therapy.

Adjuvant therapies such as gabapentin, pregabalin, ketamine, and topical agents (eg, lidocaine and capsaicin) may be beneficial in the postoperative period for pain control, but have not been studied in the elderly.[8] If adjunctive therapies are used, elderly patients should be started on a low dose that can be titrated up slowly, keeping the potential for decreased end-organ function in mind.

Nausea

Postoperative nausea and vomiting can be difficult to control in the elderly, owing to the risk of multiple ADRs with common antiemetics. Ondansetron and other serotonin receptor blockers may have fewer ADRs but should still be used cautiously in patients at risk for QTc prolongation. Use of other agents such as promethazine and prochlorperazine should be limited, owing to the level of sedation they can induce. Metoclopramide should not be used in patients with Parkinson disease because of its drug-disease interaction.[11] New agents such as aprepitant are limited by expense and multiple drug interactions. Alvimopan, which is indicated to speed the return of GI function postoperatively, is limited by its potential increased risk for myocardial infarction.

Atrial Fibrillation

The risk of atrial fibrillation increases as the body ages. The elderly may be less tolerant of tachycardia as a result of reliance on stroke volume to maintain perfusion in the setting of impaired cardiac contractility.

Unfortunately, the elderly are also not very tolerant of antiarrhythmic therapy. A post hoc analysis of the Atrial Fibrillation Follow-up Investigation of Rhythm Management (AFFIRM) trial that selected participants who were 70 to 80 years of age compared rate-control with rhythm-control therapy for atrial fibrillation. All-cause mortality was significantly lower in the rate-control group than the rhythm-control group (18% vs 23%, $P = .01$) after a median of 3.4 years of follow-up. There was no change in cardiovascular mortality, but a significant decrease in noncardiovascular mortality in the rate-control group (8% vs 12%, $P = .002$). There was also a decrease in all-cause hospitalization in the rate-control group (61% vs 68%, $P<.001$).[12] The target heart rate in this study was less than 80 beats/min at rest. A subsequent study in which the median age was 68 years found that targeting a heart rate of less than 110 beats/min instead of less than 80 beats/min decreased the composite of cardiovascular death, hospitalization due to heart failure, stroke, major bleeding, syncope, sustained ventricular tachycardia, cardiac arrest, and life-threatening adverse medication effects.[13] Both studies used β-blockers as first-line agents for rate control. In its 2011 update to the atrial fibrillation guidelines, the American Heart Association recommends that, in patients with an ejection fraction greater than 40% and no or acceptable symptoms, there is no benefit of targeting a heart rate less than 80 beats/min over targeting a heart rate less than 110 beats/min.[14]

β-Blockers and calcium-channel blockers are recommended as first-line therapy in the elderly to manage atrial fibrillation in the perioperative period. Sotalol may also be used, but must be adjusted for renal function. Digoxin is not recommended because of its multiple drug interactions and altered pharmacokinetics in the elderly. If digoxin is chosen, careful attention should be paid to the patient's renal function, as this will affect the volume of distribution of digoxin and increase the likelihood for toxicity.

Anticoagulation

Elderly patients may be at an increased risk of bleeding when initiated on anticoagulation. For patients requiring venous thromboembolism prophylaxis, time from surgery and renal function need to be considered before initiation. Many agents can be started in as little as 6 hours postoperatively. Multiple agents, however, are inappropriate for patients with renal impairment. Rivaroxaban, fondaparinux, and enoxaparin should be used with caution when estimated creatinine clearance is less than 30 mL/min. Enoxaparin in one study was also found to be associated with an increased risk of bleeding in those with a creatinine clearance between 30 and 50 mL/min.[15] Unfractionated heparin does not appear to be affected by age or renal function.

For patients who have been anticoagulated preoperatively, therapeutic anticoagulation should be restarted as soon as is safely possible. Some elderly patients will require dose adjustments to account for renal function and body weight. For example, the dose of apixaban should be reduced in patients weighing less than 60 kg to 2.5 mg twice daily, and fondaparinux should be decreased to 2.5 mg daily for weight less than 50 kg and 10 mg daily for those weighing greater than 100 kg. The newer oral anticoagulants, dabigatran, apixaban, and rivaroxaban, can generally be restarted 24 hours after surgery if there is a low bleeding risk, or in 48 to 72 hours if the bleeding risk is high.[16] The anticoagulant effect of these newer agents is seen within hours of the first dose, so they should not be concomitantly bridged with other anticoagulants.

SUMMARY

As the body ages, drug metabolism and drug effects change. These alterations in pharmacodynamics and pharmacokinetics place the elderly at an increased risk of experiencing an ADR. The incidence of medication-related adverse events can be decreased with careful selection of agents and appropriate dosage adjustments.

REFERENCES

1. Petrovic M, van der Camme T, Onder G. Adverse drug reactions in older people: detection and prevention. Drugs Aging 2012;29:453–62.
2. Pretorius RW, Gataric G, Swedlund SK, et al. Reducing the risk of adverse drug events in older adults. Am Fam Physician 2013;87:331–6.
3. Klopotowska JE, Wierenga PC, Stuijt CC, et al. Adverse drug events in older hospitalized patients: results and reliability of a comprehensive and structured identification strategy. PLoS One 2013;8:e71045. http://dx.doi.org/10.1371/journal.pone.0071045.

4. Mangoni AA, Jackson SH. Age-related changes in pharmacokinetics and pharmacodynamics: basic principles and practical applications. Br J Clin Pharmacol 2003;57:6–14.
5. Klotz U. Pharmacokinetics and drug metabolism in the elderly. Drug Metab Rev 2009;41:67–76.
6. Hubbard RE, O'Mahony MS, Woodhouse KW. Medication prescribing in frail older people. Eur J Clin Pharmacol 2013;69:319–26.
7. Mathew JP, Fontes ML, Tudor IC, et al. A multicenter risk index for atrial fibrillation after cardiac surgery. JAMA 2004;291:1720–9.
8. Schofield PA. The assessment and management of peri-operative pain in older adults. Anaesthesia 2014;69:54–60.
9. O'Neil CK, Hanlon JT, Marcum ZA. Adverse effects of analgesics commonly used by older adults with osteoarthritis: focus on non-opioid and opioid analgesics. Am J Geriatr Pharmacother 2012;10:331–42.
10. van Ojik AL, Jansen JA, Brouwers JR, et al. Treatment of chronic pain in older people. Drugs Aging 2012;29:615–25.
11. Aymanns C, Keller F, Maus S, et al. Review on pharmacokinetics and pharmacodynamics and the aging kidney. Clin J Am Soc Nephrol 2010;5:314–27.
12. Shariff N, Desai RV, Patel K, et al. Rate-control versus rhythm-control strategies and outcomes in septuagenarians with atrial fibrillation. Am J Med 2013;126: 887–93.
13. van Gelder IC, Groenveld HF, Crijns HJ, et al. Lenient versus strict rate control in patients with atrial fibrillation. N Engl J Med 2010;362:1363–73.
14. Wann LS, Curtis AB, January CT, et al. 2011 ACCF/AHA/HRS focused update on the management of patients with atrial fibrillation (updating the 2006 guidelines): a report of the American College of Cardiology Foundation/American Heart Association Task Force on Practice Guidelines. Circulation 2011;123:104–23.
15. DeCarolis DD, Thorson JG, Clarmont MA, et al. Enoxaparin outcomes in patients with moderate renal impairment. Arch Intern Med 2012;172:1713–8.
16. Spyropoulos AC, Douketis JD. How I treat anticoagulated patients undergoing an elective procedure or surgery. Blood 2012;120:2954–62.

Operative Risk Stratification in the Older Adult

Karen G. Scandrett, MD[a], Brian S. Zuckerbraun, MD[b,c], Andrew B. Peitzman, MD[c,*]

KEYWORDS

- Geriatric • Frailty • Goals of care • Cognitive function

KEY POINTS

- Older adults should undergo standard cardiopulmonary risk stratification based on history, physical, and indicated laboratory and diagnostic tests.
- Assessment of the older adult should include mental status and cognitive function evaluation.
- Functional status determination and frailty are necessary to guide decision making and true risk assessment, as well as to potentially indicate the need for "prehabilitation."
- It is necessary to define goals of care and advanced directives for older patients in the context of the current disease and their long-term prognosis.
- Overall medical care must be based on the composite of this assessment, defining personal goals, cardiopulmonary and physiologic status, functional status and frailty, and risk-to-benefit ratio.

INTRODUCTION: NATURE OF THE PROBLEM

The graying of the US population is among the most frequently described demographic shifts occurring today. The "baby boom" generation began expanding the Medicare rolls around 2010, and over the next 20 years will require more and more health care as they advance into older age. Moreover, although medical science and technology have increased life expectancy across the board, cures for many chronic medical conditions are not available, and these conditions are a source of ongoing disability and health care costs. Although disability rates have decreased modestly over the past 20 years,[1] approximately 48% of adults older than 75 years

[a] Department of Geriatric Medicine, University of Pittsburgh, Pittsburgh, PA, USA; [b] VA Pittsburgh Healthcare System, Pittsburgh, PA, USA; [c] Department of Surgery, University of Pittsburgh, Pittsburgh, PA, USA
* Corresponding author. Department of Surgery, F-1281, UPMC-Presbyterian, Pittsburgh, PA 15213.
E-mail address: peitzmanab@upmc.edu

Surg Clin N Am 95 (2015) 149–172
http://dx.doi.org/10.1016/j.suc.2014.09.014
0039-6109/15/$ – see front matter © 2015 Elsevier Inc. All rights reserved.
surgical.theclinics.com

report some physical difficulty, and 6.5% of older adults require physical assistance. As ever larger numbers of people begin aging into their 8th and 9th decades, our health care system will be under increased pressure to function more efficiently, improve outcomes, and reduce costs.[2]

Currently, hospital beds are occupied disproportionately with older adults, who in 2005 accounted for 35% of all hospitalizations despite comprising only 12% of the US population.[2] Risks of hospitalization, documented in the IOM Report *To Err is Human*,[3] are particularly high for frail older adults requiring tailored care processes.[4] Postoperative complications, for which age is an independent risk factor, increase the risk of 30-day readmission 4-fold, and the potential costs are high.[5,6] To cite 1 example, incident delirium in a hospitalized elderly patient prolongs length of stay, is associated with increased 6-month mortality, and is estimated to cost, on average, an additional $2500 per affected patient.[7]

Aging affects individuals in various ways. Some older adults remain highly functional, cognitively and physically, well into their 10th decade, whereas others may become disabled and infirm before they reach the age of 70 years. More than 80% of older adults have more than 1 chronic medical condition, and take more than 8 prescription medications.[2] Among a subset of older adults, alterations in body composition, energy balance, homeostatic regulation, and metabolism occur, which affect physiologic and functional reserve in many organ systems.[8] This phenomenon, described as frailty, is an independent predictor of poor operative risk.[9] Identification of frail patients, and those with decreased cognitive and functional reserve, is increasingly recognized as a key component of preoperative assessment in the older adult.[10]

As hospitals and health systems innovate to create safe processes and environments for their most vulnerable patients, hospital-based physicians and surgeons too must effectively utilize knowledge of how best to care for frail older adults, and quality indicators have been developed to measure and facilitate improvement in care processes for older surgical patients.[11] Geriatric assessment can guide strategies for mitigating risk during the perioperative period, and there are several models for accomplishing this. Several centers utilize perioperative geriatric consultation services among both elective and acute surgical patients, with generally positive although heterogeneous results in terms of length of stay, rates of delirium, discharge to institutional care, and 6-month mortality.[12–14] Comanagement models, in which leadership is shared between orthopedic surgery and geriatric medicine, have been shown to improve multiple outcomes for older patients with fragility fractures, including length of stay and mortality.[15,16] Although not studied in the surgical population, specialized geriatric acute care units show promise as a systems-based intervention with potential to decrease in-hospital falls, delirium, functional decline, decreased length of stay, and lower hospital costs.[17] The geriatric preoperative evaluation, described herein, presents another key opportunity to identify important concerns and address sources of increased risk.

GERIATRIC EVALUATION

Geriatric preoperative evaluation builds on preoperative evaluation in younger adults by integrating a functional orientation. "Medical clearance" for a general medical patient includes review of the medical history with a focus on cardiovascular and pulmonary health, determination of current exercise capacity, and a discussion of prior complications. Although evidence for the utility of such testing in otherwise healthy adults is lacking,[18] routine preoperative testing includes serum electrolytes, coagulation studies, a chest x-ray, and an electrocardiogram.

Geriatric preoperative evaluation extends this assessment to integrate the past and current medical conditions with the patient's overall physical function, evaluating not only the patient's operative risk, but also identifying risk factors for prolonged hospitalization and poor postoperative recovery.[19,20] In addition to the standard history and physical examination, the American College of Surgeons' *Best Practices Guideline for Optimal Preoperative Assessment of the Geriatric Surgical Patient* recommends inclusion of screening for specific geriatric syndromes[21] including cognitive and functional screening, nutritional assessment, and assessment for frailty.

HISTORY AND PHYSICAL EXAMINATION

For a patient undergoing elective or semielective surgery, there is time for a reasonably detailed discussion of past medical and surgical history, medications, and functional status. For an unstable, critically ill patient, this history may need to be gathered in parallel to or even after the life-saving procedure. In any case, each of these components of the assessment provides important information for managing the perioperative course. Moreover, often during the assessment process, cognitive limitations will emerge that signify additional postoperative risk and warrant further evaluation.

Cardiac Evaluation

Cardiac risk assessment is a well-documented aspect of preoperative assessment. The 2007 *Guideline for Perioperative Evaluation and Care for Noncardiac Surgery* from the American College of Cardiology provides a clear algorithm to determine need for further preoperative cardiac testing (**Fig. 1**).[22] Cardiac risk stratification is based on the patient's history of prior events and interventions, and an accurate report from the patient about current functional limitations. In some cases, one or both of these pieces of information may be lacking during the assessment of a frail elderly patient. In this case, a clear medical record and/or ancillary history from a collateral source can be helpful. Furthermore, age-related musculoskeletal deterioration and frailty may limit physical activity, complicating the evaluation of functional cardiac symptoms.[23] Preoperative cardiology consult may be considered in the patient with any of the following:

- Unstable angina or an acute myocardial infarction
- Decompensated heart failure
- A significant conduction defect or symptomatic arrhythmia
- Severe aortic or mitral valve disease

As indicated in the guideline, when the indication for surgery takes precedent over preoperative testing, the focus of care shifts to intraoperative and postoperative risk management.

Principles of perioperative care of the patient undergoing noncardiac surgery include:

- Continuation of β-blockers in patients who are already on β-blockers before surgery, with titration of medication to achieve a resting heart rate of 60 to 65 bpm.[24]
- Continuation of statins in patients already taking a statin.
- Management of postoperative arrhythmia, including rate control (β-blocker, calcium channel blocker, or digoxin) and treatment of underlying cause.

Older individuals are at greater risk for atrial fibrillation, ischemic heart disease, and diastolic heart failure.[25] Age-related changes in the vascular system and the myocardium result in a stiff ventricle with impaired relaxation, although decreased response to

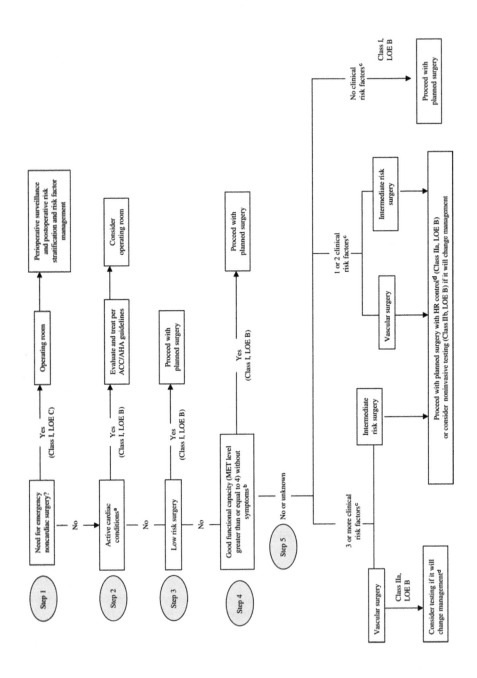

adrenergic stimulation and decreased sensitivity of the sinus node and baroreceptors decrease physiologic response to hemodynamic changes. These alterations may be relatively stable or go undetected until the patient is placed at increased stress or subjected to large volume shifts. Therefore, even in the absence of known ischemic heart disease, it is important to ascertain a history of congestive heart failure (lower extremity edema or orthopnea), to ask directly about use of a diuretic prescription, and to maintain watchfulness during the perioperative period.

Pulmonary Evaluation

Postoperative pulmonary complications occur more commonly than cardiac complications and are associated with increased cost and prolonged length of stay.[26] Pulmonary complications occur twice as often in older versus younger patients. Among older patients, pulmonary complications are associated with additional morbidities, including myocardial infarction, renal failure, venous thromboembolic disease, and perioperative and 3-month mortality. A systematic review of available evidence identified patient-related risk factors for postoperative pulmonary complications **(Table 1)**.[27]

Notably, age is independently associated with increased risk of postoperative pulmonary complications, even after adjusting for these comorbidities. This is likely related to age-related physiologic changes in pulmonary function[28] (see the article by Kaafarani, elsewhere in this issue).

Evidence does not support routine preoperative evaluation of pulmonary function. Strategies to prevent pulmonary complications include identifying patients at risk and optimizing perioperative care directed at specific risk factors.[29] These include:

- Smoking cessation
- Preoperative inspiratory muscle training
- Evaluation for undiagnosed and/or untreated obstructive sleep apnea (ie, STOP-BANG questionnaire)[30]
- Perioperative lung expansion techniques such as incentive spirometry, intermittent positive-pressure breathing, continuous positive-pressure airway pressure, and chest physiotherapy
- Anesthetic and postoperative pain management considerations, such as avoidance of longer acting neuromuscular blockade, and employment of regional anesthetic techniques.
- Surgical considerations, such as the use of minimally invasive techniques and surgical incision size and placement that minimize negative influences on respiratory mechanics.

◀──

Fig. 1. Cardiac evaluation and care algorithm for noncardiac surgery based on active clinical conditions, known cardiovascular disease, or cardiac risk factors for patients 50 years of age or greater. [a] See Table 2 for active clinical conditions. [b] See Class III recommendations in Noninvasive Stress Testing. [c] See Table 3 for estimated MET level equivalent. [d] Noninvasive testing may be considered before surgery in specific patients with risk factors if it will change management. [e] Clinical risk factors include ischemic heart disease, compensated or prior heart failure, diabetes mellitus, renal insufficiency, and cerebrovascular disease. [f] Consider perioperative β-blockade for populations in which this has been shown to reduce cardiac morbidity/mortality. ACC/AHA, American College of Cardiology/American Heart Association; HR, heart rate; LOE, level of evidence; MET, metabolic equivalent. (*From* Fleisher LA, Beckman JA, Brown KA, et al. ACC/AHA Guidelines on Perioperative Cardiovascular Evaluation and Care for Noncardiac Surgery: a report of the American College of Cardiology/American Heart Association Task Force on Practice Guidelines. J Am Coll Cardiology 2007;50(17):e159–241; with permission.)

Table 1
Patient-related risk factors for postoperative pulmonary complications

Risk Factor	Studies, n	Pooled Estimate Odds Ratio (95% CI)[a]	I^2, %[a]	Trim-and-Fill Estimate Odds Ratio (95% CI)[b]
Age (y)				
50–59	2	1.50 (1.31–1.71)	0.0	—
60–69	7	2.28 (1.86–2.80)	50.4	2.09 (1.65–2.64)
70–79	4	3.90 (2.70–5.65)	81.6	3.04 (2.11–4.39)
≥80	1	5.63 (4.63–6.85)	—	—
ASA class				
≥II[c]	6	4.87 (3.34–7.10)	0.0	4.87 (3.34–7.10)
≥III[c]	11	3.12 (2.17–4.48)	65.2	2.55 (1.73–3.76)
Abnormal chest radiograph	2	4.81 (2.43–9.55)	0.0	—
CHF	3	2.93 (1.02–8.43)	92.1	2.93 (1.02–8.03)
Arrhythmia	1	2.90 (1.10–7.50)	—	—
Functional dependence				
Partial	2	1.65 (1.36–2.01)	82.6	—
Total	2	2.51 (1.99–3.15)	67.9	—
COPD	8	2.36 (1.90–2.93)	82.0	1.79 (1.44–2.22)
Weight loss	2	1.62 (1.17–2.26)	91.7	—
Medical comorbid condition	1	1.48 (1.10–1.97)	—	—
Cigarette use	5	1.40 (1.17–1.68)	67.5	1.26 (1.01–1.56)
Impaired sensorium	2	1.39 (1.08–1.79)	63.0	—
Corticosteroid use	1	1.33 (1.12–1.58)	—	—
Alcohol use	2	1.21 (1.11–1.32)	0.0	—

Abbreviations: ASA, American Society of Anesthesiologists; CHF, congestive heart failure; COPD, chronic obstructive pulmonary disease.

[a] For I^2 definition and values, see the Appendix, available at www.annals.org.
[b] Estimates derived from meta-analysis of adjusted odds ratios from multivariable studies.
[c] When compared with patients with lower ASA class values.

From Smetana GW, Lawrence VA, Cornell JE. Preoperative pulmonary risk stratification for non-cardiothoracic surgery: Systematic review for the American College of Physicians. Ann Intern Med 2006;144(8):581–595; with permission.

Cognitive Assessment

Baseline alteration in cognitive function, both acute and chronic, places the patient at increased risk for postoperative delirium and resulting complications. Screening tools for dementia and delirium may be utilized to identify patients at risk and allow the surgery team to optimize the timing of surgery as well as provide adequate support during the perioperative period.[31]

Dementia

Dementia increases in prevalence with age, and its clinical significance ranges from subtle cognitive deficits to complete functional dependence. However, cognitive impairment is not "normal" and does not occur universally. Many older patients are cognitively intact, whereas others may present normally but have subclinical dementia that nevertheless requires vigilance for postoperative complications and increased support with the postoperative transition.

There are numerous screening tools to detect cognitive impairment and guide next steps.[32,33] The Mini-Cog is a widely used instrument that can be administered in fewer than 5 minutes in the office setting. It has high sensitivity, requires little training to administer, and is appropriate for use in a multilingual population, making it an appropriate screening tool to be used by generalists in the ambulatory setting. The instrument and its scoring algorithm are presented in **Fig. 2**.[34] An abnormal Mini-Cog assessment, obtained when the patient is at their usual baseline, indicates the presence of possible cognitive impairment and should alert providers of increased risk for postoperative delirium. A positive screen should be followed with a recommendation for a more thorough dementia evaluation when the patient's condition permits.

Delirium

Delirium is an alteration in attention and cognition that is acute in onset (having occurred within the past several hours or days) and is related to an underlying medical condition.[35] Clinical features of delirium are presented in **Table 2**.[36] Delirium is prevalent in the hospitalized elderly (estimated in approximately 30%) and is strongly associated with poor outcomes in the postoperative setting, including increased length of stay, pulmonary complications, in-hospital falls, dehydration, pressure ulcers, and urinary tract infections.[37] Risk factors for delirium can be stratified into 2 categories: Predisposing factors and precipitating factors (**Box 1**). Predisposing factors are patient

Administration:

1. Ask the patient to listen carefully to 3 unrelated words, repeat them to you, and remember them for later. You may repeat the words up to three time until they are remembered correctly.
2. Using a piece of blank paper, as the patient to draw the face of a clock and fill in all the numbers. As the patient to draw the hands to read 11:10 (or any time that utilizes both halves of the clock. Instructions may be repeated, but no additional hints.
3. Ask the patient to repeat the 3 words from before.

Scoring:

1. Give one point for each correct word to calculate recall score, maximum 3 points.
2. Score the clock normal or abnormal. (Normal: all the numbers present and in correct order and position, hands depict the correct time).
3. Determine whether screen is positive or negative for dementia using the algorithm.

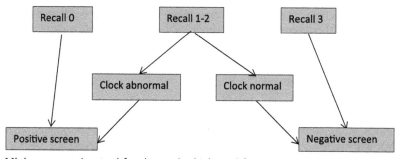

Fig. 2. Mini-cog screening tool for dementia. (*Adapted from* Borson S, Scanlan J, Brush M, et al. The mini-cog: a cognitive 'vital signs' measure for dementia screening in multi-lingual elderly. Int J Geriatr Psychiatry 2000;15(11):1021–7; with permission.)

Table 2
Clinical features of delirium: The diagnosis of delirium is made in the presence of features 1–3, and either 4 or 5

Feature Number	Feature	Description
1	Inattention	Key feature for diagnosis of delirium Difficulty focusing, and sustaining attention, maintaining conversation, following commands
2	Acute onset	Onset within hours or days Often requires reliable third party to provide history
3	Fluctuating course	Symptoms wax and wane over a 24-h period Intermittent lucid intervals are common
4	Disorganized thinking	Incoherent speech Rambling, irrelevant conversation, illogical flow of ideas
5	Altered level of consciousness	Altered awareness of the environment: Vigilant, lethargic, stupor, coma
6	Cognitive deficits	Disorientation, memory deficits, language impairment
7	Perceptual disturbances	Illusions or hallucinations
8	Psychomotor disturbances	Hyperactive: Agitation and hypervigilance Hypoactive: Lethargy, decreased motor activity Mixed
9	Sleep–wake disturbance	Daytime drowsiness, nighttime insomnia, fragmented sleep, or complete sleep cycle reversal
10	Emotional disturbance	Labile symptoms of fear, paranoia, anxiety, depression, irritability, apathy, anger, euphoria

Adapted from Inouye SK. Delirium in older persons. N Engl J Med 2006;354:1157–65.

specific; precipitating factors include intraoperative risk factors. Some precipitating factors may be modified. Treatment is of limited efficacy, but structured programs may be put utilized, which are effective in decreasing its incidence.[38–40] Strategies for treatment of delirium include those listed in **Box 2**.

Depression

Depressive symptoms are prevalent among older adults, affecting up to 16% of the community-dwelling elderly, 25% of older patients in primary care settings, and 50% to 70% of long-term care residents. Although rates of major depression are lower than in young populations, depressive symptoms can be psychosocially debilitating to older adults, and are associated with increased morbidity and health care utilization.[42] The presence of depression may adversely impact postoperative recovery, and has been associated with:

- Increased pain perception and need for increased analgesia[43]
- Poor functional recovery[44]
- Increased mortality after cardiac surgery[45]

Although there are multiple effective treatment modalities for depression, many cases go undetected or untreated owing to the presence of other cognitive disorders and/or stigma associated with diagnosis. Therefore, screening for depression is appropriate and may improve long term outcomes, when linked to appropriate follow-up and ongoing care.[46] Although multiple screening tools exist, the Patient Health Questionnaire-2 is recommended as a brief and reliable, validated screen for

Box 1
Risk factors for delirium

Predisposing Factors

Demographics

　Age

　Male sex

Cognitive status

　Dementia

　Delirium

　Depression

Functional status

　Dependence

　Immobility

　Low activity

　Falls

Sensory impairment

　Visual

　Hearing

Decreased intake

　Dehydration

　Malnutrition

Drugs

　Psychoactive medications

　Polypharmacy

　Ethyl alcohol

Comorbidity

　Severe illness

　Multiple conditions

　Chronic kidney or liver disease

　Cerebrovascular accident

　Neurologic

　Metabolic derangements

　Trauma

　Terminal illness

　Human immunodeficiency virus

Precipitating Factors

Drugs

　Sedative/hypnotics

　Narcotics

　Anticholinergic medications

Polypharmacy

Ethyl alcohol withdrawal

Primary neurologic disease

Stroke

Intracranial hemorrhage

Meningitis

Intercurrent illness

Infection

Iatrogenic complications

Severe illness

Hypoxia

Shock

Fever

Anemia

Dehydration

Poor nutrition

Metabolic derangement

Surgery

Orthopedic

High-risk surgery

Prolonged bypass

Emergency surgery

Environmental

Intensive care unit admission

Use of restraints

Bladder catheter

Multiple procedures

Uncontrolled pain

Emotional stress

Sleep deprivation

Predisposing factors include patient characteristics or preexisting conditions, whereas precipitating factors relate to the current situation or acute event.

depression that can be performed in the office setting (**Fig. 3**).[47,48] A positive screen should be followed by consultation with the primary care physician, geriatrician, or mental health professional for further evaluation and development of a treatment plan.

Substance abuse

Alcohol is the primary substance abused by the elderly population. In a 2005–2006 national survey, 13% of men and 8% of women age 65 and older reported at-risk drinking (14 drinks per week for men, 7 drinks per week for women).[49] Moreover,

---
Box 2
Strategies for treatment of delirium

- Perioperative geriatric consultations to identify higher risk patients and recommend targeted preventive strategies.

- Lighter anesthetic regimens, such as titrating anesthetic agents, to maintain bispectral index (BIS) between 40 and 60 and avoiding episodes of deep anesthesia (BIS <40).

- Maintenance of sleep–wake cycles using bright light therapy.

- Hospital Elder Life Program consisting of early mobilization, behavioral measures to promote sleep and orientation, communication methods and adaptive equipment, and early intervention for dehydration.

- Provision of adequate analgesia.

- Avoidance of benzodiazepines and antihistamines[41] (unless needed to treat ethyl alcohol withdrawal).

- Use of low dose antipsychotics (eg, haloperidol 0.5 mg every 6 hours) may reduce duration of symptoms.

---

age-related changes in body composition result in greater blood alcohol concentration per amount consumed. Alcohol abuse may be missed in older adults because of reduced social and occupational interaction, and more often presents as poor self-care, nutritional deficiency, or medical illness.[50] In addition to greater risk for withdrawal syndromes, older patients with alcohol dependency are at high risk for hospital complications, including pneumonia, sepsis, surgical site infection, wound disruption, and longer length of stay. For these reasons it is important to screen for alcohol use preoperatively. The CAGE questionnaire (**Fig. 4**) is a time-tested screening tool that is brief and effective and performs well in the elderly population.[51] Patients with a positive screen should receive folate and thiamine supplementation and be evaluated frequently for withdrawal symptoms.

Nutritional Assessment

Nutritional status is an independent risk factor for postoperative recovery and a recognized quality indicator both for preoperative assessment of the older surgical patient and for general care of the hospitalized older patient. Although no gold standard indicator of nutritional status has been established, some commonly used measures include:

- Serum albumin or prealbumin
- Total cholesterol
- Body mass index less than 22
- Unintentional weight loss
- Specific vitamin deficiencies (eg, B_{12}, folate)

Of these, a recent systematic review identified serum albumin and unintentional weight loss of greater than 10% in the previous 6 months to be the best predictors of postoperative complications.[52] A positive screen for any of these factors should be followed by a full nutritional assessment and implementation of a preoperative nutritional plan. The plan may include liberalizing a restrictive diet to increase caloric or protein intake, provision of nutritional supplements, and addressing comorbid conditions and medications impacting intake and appetite.[53] Although not specifically studied in the geriatric population, there may be a benefit of brief preoperative immunonutrition therapy.[54]

Over the past two weeks, how often have you been bothered by any of the following problems?

Little interest or pleasure in doing things.
0 = Not at all
1 = Several days
2 = More than half the days
3 = Nearly every day

Feeling down, depressed, or hopeless.
0 = Not at all
1 = Several days
2 = More than half the days
3 = Nearly every day

Total point score: _____

Score interpretation:

PHQ-2 score	Probability of major depressive disorder (%)	Probability of any depressive disorder (%)
1	15.4	36.9
2	21.1	48.3
3	38.4	75.0
4	45.5	81.2
5	56.4	84.6
6	78.6	92.9

Fig. 3. Patient health questionnaire 2 (PHQ-2). (*From* Kroenke K, Spitzer RL, Williams JB. The patient health questionnaire-2: validity of a two-item depression screener. Med Care 2003;41(11):1284–92; with permission.)

In addition, geriatric surgical patients are at greater risk for dysphagia during the postoperative period. Most of the time, age-related slowing in swallowing function does not increase the risk for aspiration. However, during the perioperative period some compensatory mechanisms may be blunted owing to delirium (from medication, alteration in day/night cycles, concomitant infection, or stress of illness) or to postoperative laryngeal swelling.[55,56] Once aware of these risks, surgical and nursing staff may take steps to modify the diet consistency, and to ensure optimal upright

Answering yes to two or more questions indicates probable alcohol abuse

C : Have you ever felt that you should **C**ut down on your drinking?

A: Have people **A**nnoyed you by criticizing your drinking?

G: Have you ever felt bad or **G**uilty about your drinking?

E: Have you ever had a drink as an **E**ye-opener first thing in the morning to steady your nerves or help a hangover?

Fig. 4. CAGE screening assessment for alcohol abuse. (*Adapted from* Buchsbaum DG, Buchanan RG, Welsh J, et al. Screening for drinking disorders in the elderly using the CAGE questionnaire. J Am Geriatr Soc 1992;40(7):662–5; with permission.)

positioning during ingestion. Speech therapy evaluation and treatment can be helpful, especially after a prolonged intensive care unit stay or endotracheal intubation. It is important to be mindful that the change in texture and palatability of modified diets may create another barrier to adequate nutritional intake.

Functional Assessment

Preoperative function has been shown to predict postoperative recovery,[44] and together with comorbidity and frailty to be predictive of mortality.[57,58] Therefore, it is important to adequately assess and communicate about this domain. Discussion of the patient's functional baseline may prompt exploration of desired functional outcome from surgery, and aid in establishing goals of care. Functional screening questions include identification of need for assistance with basic and instrumental activities of daily living (**Box 3**). Further questions may assess whether any limitations are related to pain/physical symptoms or to cognitive issues. A person's functional status

---

Box 3
Basic and instrumental activities of daily living

Basic Activities of Daily Living

Dressing

Bathing

Eating

Continence

Transfer

Ambulation

Instrumental Activities of Daily Living

Cooking

Shopping

Transportation

Finances

Telephone

Housekeeping

---

may be obvious when the patient has clearly identified needs for basic assistance and resides in a long term care facility, but may be more difficult to gauge in those who are just "getting by" in their home environments.

Frailty

Frailty is a multidimensional concept that describes decreased physiologic and functional reserve. Although frailty is a widely recognized phenomenon, it was first described in the medical literature by Fried in 2001. Components of the phenotype include:

- Shrinking and weight loss
- Poor endurance or exhaustion
- Weakness
- Slow walking speed
- Low physical activity level

Frailty is distinct from, but overlaps with, disability and comorbidity, and has been investigated as a surgical risk assessment tool. Frailty is associated with longer postoperative recovery, discharge to a nursing facility, prolonged rehabilitation, and increased 6-month and 1-year mortality in comparison with age-adjusted controls.[9,59]

Multiple instruments have been developed to assess frailty in the clinical setting.[60] There is no uniform definition of frailty, but many of the instruments developed build on the description of the frailty phenotype that was established through population research. Components of the frailty phenotype can be assessed using validated instruments (**Table 3**). Some instruments also measure additional domains including cognition and social support.[61] Other groups utilize accumulated deficits models that incorporate frailty characteristics, including symptoms, signs, disabilities, diseases, and laboratory values.[59,62,63] Although many tools have been developed for research purposes, there is a lack of consensus about the best way to assess frailty in the office setting.

Table 3		
Assessment for phenotypic frailty		
Frailty Factor	**Measure**	**Notes**
Shrinking	Unintentional weight loss of >10 lb	Self-report
Weakness	Decreased grip strength	Three trials using handheld dynamometer with dominant hand, result adjusted by gender and body mass index
Exhaustion	Center for Epidemiologic Studies – Depression scale (CES-D)	"I felt everything I did was an effort" or "I could not get going" a moderate amount or most of the time
Slowness	Gait speed	Three trials of walking 15 ft at a normal pace, result adjusted for gender and height
Low activity	Minnesota Leisure Time Activities Questionnaire	Weekly tasks converted to equivalent kilocalories; total expenditure adjusted for gender

The frailty phenotype is defined by 5 factors, which may be assessed using standardized instruments.
Adapted from Makary MA, Segev DL, Pronovost PJ, et al. Frailty as a predictor of surgical outcomes in older patients. J Am Coll Surg 2010;210:901–8; with permission.

Multiple studies have demonstrated that frailty is a reliable surgical risk indicator. Preoperative frailty was associated with increased postoperative complications, longer hospital stays, and higher 30-day readmission rates,[64,65] and with discharge to a skilled or assisted living facility after living at home.[9] Of note, frailty assessments have been shown to outperform traditional risk assessment tools, and have had an additive value in combining with other scoring systems such as the American Society of Anesthesiology Physical Status Classification System score or the Eagle Criteria for cardiac risk.[66]

In addition to using frailty for risk stratification, ultimately this concept may be used to determine the need for interventions among patients diagnosed as frail. One group used a bundled intervention to prevent functional decline that is similar to the approach used in delirium prevention, and achieved a reduction in frailty at the time of hospital discharge.[67] Additional proposed "prehabilitation" strategies include nutritional and/or exercise interventions to counteract sarcopenia, or replacement of testosterone in hypogonadal older men.[68,69]

Medication Review

Medication review in the geriatric surgical patient begins with an accurate listing of all medications that are being taken by the patient, including prescription medication, over-the-counter medications, and herbal or alternative therapies. Because older patients may take a large number of medications, they are at greater risk for both drug–drug interactions and drug–disease interactions. Many medications are safely held during surgery and postoperatively, but some, including β-blockers, are best to be continued. Others, such as oral anticoagulants or antiplatelet agents, may require additional care and communication with regard to timing of surgery or to resumption of medication postoperatively. Still others, such as maintenance steroids, benzodiazepines, or antiseizure medications, may precipitate harmful symptoms if discontinued abruptly, and consideration should be given to continuing them at a low dose. Consultation with the hospital pharmacist can be helpful in completing an accurate medication reconciliation for higher risk patients, and identifying potential medication-related adverse events.

Beers Criteria

The well-known Beers criteria for potentially inappropriate medication use in older adults were updated in 2012.[70] Despite the widespread recognition of the Beers criteria, and uptake of these recommendations into policy and quality measures, many of the listed medications are still being prescribed to older adults. The process for updating the Beers criteria included a review and grading of new evidence underpinning each recommendation. As with the prior criteria, recommendations are divided into 2 categories: (1) Potentially inappropriate medications for any older adult, and (2) medications with potential for drug–disease or drug–syndrome interaction. A select list of potentially inappropriate medications is displayed in **Table 4**.

Cardiac Medications

Perioperative cardiovascular care guidelines have provided direction with regard to cardiac medication use.[21] This guidance includes maintaining perioperative β-blockade in patients already on this medication, and recommends against routine β-blocker initiation in patients not currently taking this class of medication.[24] Treatment should be titrated to optimize blood pressure and avoid bradycardia. Because older adults with multiple medical comorbidities have often been excluded from the clinical trials that inform evidence-based guidelines, adherence to guidelines should

Table 4
Beers criteria: potentially inappropriate medications for use with older adults

Therapeutic Category	Selected Drugs	Rationale/Comments
Systemic		
Antihistamines	Diphenhydramine, hydroxyzine, promethazine, chlorpheniramine	Highly anticholinergic, clearance reduced with advanced age
Antiparkinson agents	Benztropine, trihexyphenidyl	More effective agents available for prevention of EPS
Antispasmodics	Dicyclomine, hyoscyamine, scopolamine	Highly anticholinergic, uncertain effectiveness
Antithrombotics	Short acting dipyridamole	Orthostasis; acceptable for use in cardiac testing
Anti-infective	Nitrofurantoin	Potential for pulmonary toxicity; lack of efficacy in CrCl <60 mL/min
Cardiovascular		
Alpha 1 blockers	Doxazosin, prazosin, terazosin	Orthostasis
Alpha agonists, central	Clonidine	Adverse CNS effects, bradycardia, orthostasis
Antiarrythmics	Flecainide, propafenone, sotalol, etc Amiodarone Dronederone Digoxin >0.125 Nifedipine	Rate control yields better balance of benefit/harm Amiodarone toxicity Worse outcomes in patients with AF or CHF No additional benefit with higher dose Potential for hypotension
Diuretics	Spironolactone	Higher risk of hyperkalemia Avoid in CrCl <30 mL/min
CNS		
Tertiary tricyclic antidepressants	Amitriptyline, doxepin, imipramine	Anticholinergic, sedation, orthostasis
Antipsychotics, all first and second generation	Haldol, chlorpromazine, olanzapine, quetiapine, risperidone, aripiprazole Thioridizine, mesoridazine	Increased risk of CVA and mortality, try nonpharmacologic measures first Risk of QT prolongation
Barbiturates	Phenobarbital, butalbital	Tolerance, physical dependence
Benzodiazipines, short and intermediate Benzodiazepine, long acting	Alprazolam, lorazepam, temazepam, triazolam, etc Clonazepam, diazepam, etc	Increased sensitivity and slower metabolism in older adults. Risk for cognitive impairment, delirium, injuries. May be appropriate in certain clinical circumstances: Seizure disorder, withdrawal, anesthesia, end of life.
Nonbenzodiazepine hypnotics	Zolpidem, eszopiclone	Benzodiazepine-receptor agonists, similar adverse events to above, lack of efficacy

Endocrine		
Hormonal agents	Testosterone, methyltestosterone	Potential for cardiac problems, contraindicated in prostate cancer
	Desicated thyroid	Cardiac effects
	Estrogens, oral and topical patch	Carcinogenic potential, no beneficial cardiac or cognitive effect Use of low dose vaginal cream is acceptable
	Megestrol	Minimal effect on weight. Prothrombotic, associated with increased mortality
	Growth hormone	Small desired effect. Adverse effects: edema, arthralgia, carpal tunnel, gynecomastia, impaired fasting glucose
Insulin	Sliding scale	Higher risk of hypoglycemia without benefit
Long acting sulfonylureas	Chlorpropamide, glyburide	Prolonged half-life, prolonged hypoglycemia, SIADH
Gastrointestinal	Metoclopramide	EPS, tardive dyskinesia
	Mineral oil	Potential for aspiration
Analgesics		
Narcotics	Meperidine	Not effective, may cause neurotoxicity
	Pentazocine	Causes confusion, hallucinations
Non–COX-selective NSAIDs	Aspirin, diclofenac, ibuprofen, ketorolac, meloxicam, naproxen, piroxicam, sulindac, etc	Increase risk of GI bleeding PPI or misoprostol reduces but does not eliminate risk
	Indomethacin	Highest risk NSAID
Skeletal muscle relaxants	Cyclobenzaprine, carisoprodol, orphenadrine, etc	Anticholinergic. Sedation and confusion

Abbreviations: AF, atrial fibrillation; CHF, congestive heart failure; CNS, central nervous system; COX, cyclooxygenase; CrCl, creatinine clearance; CVA, cerebrovascular accident; EPS, extrapyramidal symptoms; GI, gastrointestinal; NSAID, nonsteroidal anti-inflammatory drug; PPI, proton pump inhibitor; SIADH, syndrome of inappropriate antidiuretic hormone.

Adapted from American Geriatrics Society 2012 Beers Criteria Update Expert Panel. American Geriatrics Society updated Beers criteria for potentially inappropriate medication use in older adults. J Am Geriatr Soc 2012;60(4):616–31.

be thoughtful.[71] For example, the HYVET trial established a treatment target blood pressure of 150/80 mm Hg in the older population (less restrictive than for younger patients), demonstrating reduced risk of congestive heart failure, death from stroke, and all-cause mortality.[72] Medical management for heart failure, more prevalent in older patients, should be tailored to optimize symptom control and minimize adverse medication events when considering guideline recommendations.[25]

Anticoagulation management can be challenging in older patients. Meta-analyses of newer anticoagulants such as gabitraban, apixiban, and rivaroxaban have demonstrated modest improvement in risk of stroke and venous thromboembolism, with no change in the risk of major bleeding.[73] However, multiple clinical questions persist with regard to these agents, including use in valvular heart disease, rebound hypercoagulability, and optimal management of bleeding complications; widespread uptake has not yet occurred.[74] Oral anticoagulation with warfarin can be complicated by nutritional deficiency, drug–drug interactions (including perioperative antibiotics), and age-related alteration in pharmacokinetics; therefore, among older patients it is recommended to use a lower dose initiation regimen when the baseline dose is not known.

In summary, recommendations for perioperative cardiac medications include:

- Continuation of preoperative β-blocker
- Close monitoring of volume status with judicious use of diuretic agents
- Lower dose warfarin initiation, with no more than 5 mg given initially

PATIENT PREFERENCE

Discussion with the patient and his or her surrogates about surgical risk and benefit is central to the preoperative evaluation. Appropriate care for older adults should take into account the priorities of the patient, as well as their overall prognosis, when determining an optimal care plan.[75,76] Communication models may help to frame the role of the physician or surgeon in this regard.[77]

Decisional Capacity

As a first step, the surgery team must determine whether the patient has capacity to engage in the decision-making process, and if not, must identify who the surrogate decision maker is. Capacity is specific to the decision; the higher the stakes of the decision, the more important that the patient or surrogate understands the nuances of the deliberation. The preoperative functional assessment will help the surgeon to understand whether the patient is operating independently, or is supported by family or others for instrumental support. Dependence in these domains suggests the need to involve a health care agent in the discussion.

Shared Decision Making

A communication model displaying a range of physician and patient roles is displayed in **Table 5**. In some instances, the need for surgery is urgent and imminent, and the goal of discussion is to communicate about surgical risk and most likely range of outcomes. In this case, the surgeon will take a more directive role in the discussion. In contrast, some clinical situations have greater latitude. Shared decision making provides a framework for the practitioner and the patient to deliberate over potential interventions in situations that are more preference sensitive, such as early stage breast cancer, low back pain, stable coronary artery disease, or prostate cancer.[78] Condition-specific decision aids have been developed to facilitate this process,[79] which allows the values and preferences of the patient to emerge. In shared decision making, the surgeon plays a more interpretive or collaborative role in the conversation.

Table 5
Models for medical decision-making. The physician's role in communication may vary depending on the clinical situation

Model	Patient Values/Goals	Physician Role
Informed consent	Known and articulated by patient	Technical expert: Provides information and implements choice
Interpretive	Unknown or conflicted	Advisor: Elucidates and interprets values, provides information and implements choice
Collaborative	Develops through discussion	Teacher: Articulates choices, provides and interprets information, persuades and implements choice
Paternalism	Imposed by physician	Guardian: Promotes the patient's well-being independent of patient preference

Adapted from Emanuel EJ, Emanuel LL. Four models of the physician-patient relationship. JAMA 1992;267(16):2221–6.

Principles for caring for older adults with multiple comorbidities have been developed by the American Geriatric Society[80] (**Table 6**), and may be used to guide discussion in the preoperative setting. Informed by patient values and preferences, decisions are based on the risks and benefits of the operation, prognosis from the disease for which the operation is being considered, and the impact on the patient's overall health condition. Functional and cognitive status, degree of comorbidity, frailty, and overall life expectancy frame the likelihood of attaining the patient's desired outcome.[81] Sometimes, alternate surgical approaches may be discussed that are more likely to achieve a patient's particular goal (such as choosing a palliative rather than a curative resection).[82]

Table 6
Guiding principles for the care of older adults with multimorbidity

Guiding Principle	Parameters to Consider
Elicit patient preferences	What is the clinical situation, and what are the patient's objectives? What personal and cultural values inform this discussion?
Interpret evidence	To what extent were older adults included in the evidence base? Does the outcome apply to this patient's particular condition? Will the treatment exacerbate another condition?
Estimate prognosis	What are the risks, burdens, and benefits of this treatment? What is this patient's life expectancy, functional status, and quality of life?
Determine clinical feasibility	What is the anticipated burden from this treatment? How will it impact other medical conditions and functional status?
Prioritize the care plan	Is this a priority procedure? How can it optimize benefit, minimize harm, and enhance quality of life?

Adapted from American Geriatric Society Expert Panel on the Care of Older Adults with Multimorbidity. Patient-centered care for older adults with multiple chronic conditions: a stepwise approach from the American Geriatrics Society. J Am Geriatr Soc 2012;60(10):1957–68.

Tools have been developed to assist with prognostication.[83,84] For patients of very advanced age who are weighing the risks and benefits of an elective operation, or their caregivers, population-based data about life expectancy are available in a web-based format that can provide an individualized estimate.[85] Additional resources are available to help determine the risk of a given operation based on the likelihood of surgical complications or morbidity, such as the American College of Surgeons Surgical Risk Calculator.[86] The estimations from this tool are calculated using data from a large number of patients who underwent a surgical procedure similar to the one the patient may have, and are based on information provided about the patient's previous history and health status. Along with clear information about the risks of surgery, and expectations for the recovery period that are based on the patient's preoperative functional status, this information may help to frame a discussion that is tailored to the patient's desired outcome.

SUMMARY

Preoperative assessment of the geriatric patient differs from general preoperative assessment by taking a functional approach. Although some older patients may be in excellent health, others may have cognitive and/or functional limitations that put them at greater risk for postoperative complications, longer length of stay, and increased morbidity and mortality. In addition, many older patients are on multiple medications and have multiple comorbidities that increase their risk for adverse medication-related events. Appropriate preoperative assessment will identify those who are at greater risk for poor outcomes, enabling the surgeon and patient to have an informed discussion about their risk. Furthermore, knowledge of preoperative functional and cognitive limitations and nutritional deficits allows the treating team to provide appropriate hospital care. Many of the assessments described herein may be performed by members of the surgical team other than the attending surgeon. However, it is the role of the surgeon to integrate the information gained from these multiple sources in order to direct a treatment plan that safely and most effectively meets the patient's goal.

REFERENCES

1. Fries JF, Bruce B, Chakravasky E. Compression of morbidity 1980-2011. J Aging Res 2011;2011:261702. http://dx.doi.org/10.4061/2011/261702.
2. Institute of Medicine (IOM). Retooling for an aging America: building the health care workforce. Washington, DC: National Academy Press; 2008.
3. Institute of Medicine (IOM). To err is human: building a safer health system. Washington, DC: National Academy Press; 2000.
4. Arora VM, Johnson M, Olson J, et al. Using acute care of vulnerable elderly quality indicators to measure the quality of hospital care for vulnerable elders. J Am Geriatr Soc 2007;55:1705–11.
5. Glance LG, Kellermann AL, Osler TM, et al. Hospital readmission after noncardiac surgery: the role of major complications. JAMA Surg 2014. http://dx.doi.org/10.1001/jamasurg.2014.4.
6. Sieber FE, Barnett SR. Preventing postoperative complications in the elderly. Anesthesiol Clin 2011;29:83–97.
7. Rubin FH, Neal K, Fenlon K. Sustainability and Scalability of the Hospital Elder Life Program at a Community Hospital. J Am Geriatr Soc 2011;59:359–65.
8. Fried LP, Tangen CM, Walston J, et al. Frailty in older adults: evidence for a phenotype. J Gerontol A Biol Sci Med Sci 2001;56(3):M146–56.

9. Makary MA, Segev DL, Pronovost PJ, et al. Frailty as a predictor of surgical outcomes in older patients. J Am Coll Surg 2010;210:901–8.
10. Zenilman M. Geriatric surgery: past, present and future. Arch Surg 2012;147:10.
11. McGory ML, Kao KK, Shekelle PG. Developing quality indicators for elderly surgical patients. Ann Surg 2009;250:338–47.
12. Partridge JS, Harari D, Martin FC, et al. The impact of pre-operative comprehensive geriatric assessment on postoperative outcomes in older patients undergoing scheduled surgery: a systematic review. Anaesthesia 2014;69:8–16.
13. Lenartowicz M, Parkovnick M, McRarlan A, et al. An evaluation of a proactive geriatric trauma consultation service. Ann Surg 2012;256:1098–101.
14. Deschodt M, Flamain J, Haentjens P, et al. Impact of geriatric consultation teams on clinical outcome in acute hospitals: a systematic review and meta-analysis. BMC Med 2013;11:48.
15. Liem IS, Kammerlander C, Suhm N, et al. Literature review of outcome parameters used in studies of geriatric fracture centers. Arch Orthop Trauma Surg 2014; 134:181–7.
16. Grigoryan KV, Javedan H, Rudolph JL. Orthogeriatric care models and outcomes in hip fracture patients: a systematic review and meta-analysis. J Orthop Trauma 2014;28:e49–55.
17. Fox MT, Persaud M, Maimets I, et al. Effectiveness of acute geriatric unit care using acute care for elders components: a systematic review and meta-analysis. J Am Geriatr Soc 2012;60:2237–45.
18. Johansson T, Fritsch G, Flamm M, et al. Effectiveness of non-cardiac preoperative testing in non-cardiac elective surgery: a systematic review. Br J Anaesth 2013;110(6):926–39. http://dx.doi.org/10.1093/bja/aet071.
19. Kabarriti AE, Pietzak EJ, Canter DJ, et al. The relationship between age and perioperative complications. Curr Geri Rep 2014;3:8–13.
20. Bettelli G. Preoperative evaluation in geriatric surgery: comorbidity, functional status and pharmacological history. Minerva Anestesiol 2011;77:637–46.
21. Chow WB, Rosenthal RA, Merkow RP, et al. Optimal preoperative assessment of the geriatric surgical patient: a best practices guideline from the American College of Surgeons National Surgical Quality Improvement Program and the American Geriatrics Society. J Am Coll Surg 2012;215(4):453–66.
22. Fleisher LA, Beckman JA, Brown KA, et al. ACC.AHA 2007 guidelines on perioperative cardiovascular evaluation and care for noncardiac surgery: a report of the ACC/AHA task force on practice guidelines. J Am Coll Cardiol 2007;50: e159–241.
23. Afilalo J, Alexander KP, Mack MJ. Frailty assessment in cardiovascular care of older adults. J Am Coll Cardiol 2014;63(8):747–62.
24. Fleischman KE, Beckman JA, Buller CE, et al. 2009 ACCF/AHA Focused update on perioperative beta blockade. J Am Coll Cardiol 2009;54(22):2102–28.
25. Rich MW. Heart failure in the 21st century: a cardiogeriatric syndrome. J Gerontol A Biol Sci Med Sci 2001;56(2):M88–96.
26. Shander A, Fleisher LA, Baria PS, et al. Clinical and economic burden of postoperative pulmonary complications: patient safety summit on definition, risk reducing interventions, and preventive strategies. Crit Care Med 2011;39(9): 2163–72.
27. Smetana GW, Lawrence VA, Cornell JE. Preoperative pulmonary risk stratification for noncardiothoracic surgery: systematic review for the American College of Physicians. Ann Intern Med 2006;144(8):581–95.
28. Chan ED, Welsh CH. Geriatric respiratory medicine. Chest 1998;114:1704–33.

29. Qaseem A, Snow V, Fitterman N, et al. Risk assessment for a strategies to reduce perioperative pulmonary complications for patients undergoing noncardiothoracic surgery: a guideline from the American college of physicians. Ann Intern Med 2006;144(8):575–80.

30. Shahid A, Wilkinson K, Marcu S, et al. STOP-Band Questionaire in STOP, THAT and 100 other sleep scales. New York: Springer; 2012. p. 373–83.

31. Robinson TN, Wu DS, Pointer LF, et al. Preoperative cognitive dysfunction is related to adverse postoperative outcomes in the elderly. J Am Coll Surg 2012; 215:12–8.

32. Lin JS, Oconnor E, Rossom RC, et al. Screening for cognitive impairment in older adults: a systematic review for the U.S. Preventive Services Task Force. Ann Intern Med 2013;159(9):601–12.

33. Brodaty H, Low LF, Gibson L, et al. What is the best dementia screening instrument for general practitioners to use? Am J Geriatr Psychiatry 2006;14(5):391–400.

34. Borson S, Scanlan J, Brush M, et al. The mini-cog: a cognitive 'vital signs' measure for dementia screening in multi-lingual elderly. Int J Geriatr Psychiatry 2000; 15(11):1021–7.

35. Inouye SK. Delirium in older persons. N Engl J Med 2006;354:1157–65.

36. Inouye SK, Van Dyck CH, Alessi CA, et al. Clarifying confusion: The Confusion Assessment Method. A new method for detection of delirium. Ann Intern Med 1990;113:941–8.

37. Rudolph JL, Marcantonio ER. Postoperative delirium: acute change with long term implications. Anesth Analg 2011;112(5):1202–11. http://dx.doi.org/10.1213/ANE.0b013e3182147f6d.

38. Moyce A, Rodseth RN, Biccard BM. The efficacy of peri-operative interventions to decreased postoperative delirium in non-cardiac surgery: a systematic review and meta-analysis. Anaesthesia 2014;69:259–69.

39. Inouye SK, Bogardu ST, Charpentie PA, et al. A multicomponent intervention to prevent delirium in hospitalized older patients. N Engl J Med 1999;340: 669–76.

40. Marcantonio ER, Flacker JM, Wright RJ, et al. Reducing delirium after hip fracture: a randomized trial. J Am Geriatr Soc 2001;49:516–22.

41. Clegg A, Young JB. Which medications to avoid in people at risk of delirium: a systematic review. Age Ageing 2011;40:23–9.

42. Ellison JM, Kyomen HH, Harper DG. Depression in later life: an overview with treatment recommendations. Psychiatr Clin North Am 2012;35:203–29. http://dx.doi.org/10.1016/j.psc.2012.01.003.

43. Taenzer P, Melzack R, Jeans ME. Influence of psychological factors on postoperative pain, mood and analgesic requirements. Pain 1986;24:331–42.

44. Lawrence VA, Hazuda HP, Cornell JE, et al. Functional independence after major abdominal surgery in the elderly. J Am Coll Surg 2004;199(5):762–72.

45. Ho PM, Masoudi FA, Spertus JA, et al. Depression predicts mortality following cardiac valve surgery. Ann Thorac Surg 2005;79:1255–9.

46. Pignone MP, Gaynes BN, Rushton JL, et al. Screening for depression in adults: a summary of the evidence for the U.S. Preventive Services Task Force. Ann Intern Med 2002;136:765–76.

47. Kroenke K, Spitzer RL, Williams JB. The Patient Health Questionnaire-2: validity of a two-item depression screener. Med Care 2003;41:1284–92.

48. Li C, Friedman B, Conwell Y, et al. Validity of the Patient Health Questionnaire 2 (PHQ-2) in identifying major depression in older people. J Am Geriatr Soc 2007;55:596–602.

49. Blazer DG, Wu LT. The epidemiology of at-risk and binge drinking among middle-aged and elderly community adults: National Survey on Drug Use and Health. Am J Psychiatry 2009;166(10):1162–9. http://dx.doi.org/10.1176/appi.ajp.2009.09010016.

50. Wartenberg AA, Nirenberg TD. Alcohol and other drug abuse in older patients. In: Gallo JJ, editor. Reichel's care of the elderly. 5th edition. Philadelphia: Lippincott Williams and Wilkins; 1999. p. 133–41.

51. Buchsbaum DG, Buchanan RG, Welsh J, et al. Screening for drinking disorders in the elderly using the CAGE questionnaire. J Am Geriatr Soc 1992;40(7):662–5.

52. Van Stign MR, Korkic-Halilovic I, Bakker M, et al. Preoperative nutrition status and postoperative outcome in elderly general surgery patients: a systematic review. JPEN Parenter Enteral Nutr 2013;37:37–43.

53. Vellas B, Lauque S, Andrieu S, et al. Nutritional assessment in the elderly. Current Opinion in Clinical Nutrition and Metablic Care 2001;4:5–8.

54. Tepaske R, Velthuis te H, Oudemans-vanStraaten HM, et al. The effect of preoperative oral immune-enhancing nutrition supplements on patients at high risk of infection after cardiac surgery: a randomized placebo-controlled trial. Lancet 2001;358:696–701.

55. Marik PE, Kaplan D. Aspiration pneumonia and dysphagia in the elderly. Chest 2003;124:328–36.

56. Langmore SE, Terpenning MS, Schork A, et al. Predictors of aspiration pneumonia: how important is dysphagia? Dysphagia 1998;13:69–81.

57. Robinson TN, Eiseman B, Wallace JI, et al. Redefining geriatric preoperative assessment using frailty, disability and co-morbidity. Ann Surg 2009;250:449–55.

58. Hamel MG, Henderson WG, Khuri SF, et al. Surgical outcomes for patients ages 80 and older: morbidity and mortality from major noncardiac surgery. J Am Geriatr Soc 2005;53:424–9.

59. Saxton A, Velanovich V. Preoperative frailty and quality of life as predictors of postoperative complications. Ann Surg 2011;253:1223–9.

60. De Vries NM, Staal JB, van Ravensberg CD, et al. Outcome instruments to measure frailty: a systematic review. Ageing Res Rev 2011;10:104–14.

61. Rothman MA, Leo-Summers L, Gill TM. Prognostic significance of potential frailty criteria. J Am Geriatr Soc 2008;56:2211–6.

62. Rockwood KM. Long-term risks of death and institutionalization of elderly people in relation to deficit accumulation at age 70. J Am Geriatr Soc 2006;54:975–9.

63. Jones DM, Song X, Rockwood K. Operationalizing a frailty index from a standardized comprehensive geriatric assessment. J Am Geriatr Soc 2004;52:1929–33.

64. Revenig LM, Canter DJ, Taylor MD. Too frail for surgery? Initial results of a large multidisciplinary prospective study examining preoperative variables predictive of poor surgical outcomes. J Am Coll Surg 2013;217:665–70.

65. Robinson TN. Simple frailty score predicts postoperative complications across surgical specialties. Am J Surg 2013;206:544–50.

66. Farhat JS, Velanovich V, Falvo AJ, et al. Are the frail destined to fail? Frailty index as predictor of surgical morbidity and mortality in the elderly. J Trauma Acute Care Surg 2012;72:1526–31.

67. Chen CC, Chen CN, Lai I, et al. Effects of a modified hospital elderlife program on frailty in individuals undergoing major elective abdominal surgery. J Am Geriatr Soc 2014;62:261–8.

68. Partridge JS, Harari D, Dhesi JK. Frailty in the older surgical patient: a review. Age Ageing 2012;41:142–7.

69. Revenig LM, Ogan K, Guzzo TJ, et al. The use of frailty as a surgical risk assessment tool in elderly patients. Curr Geriatr Rep 2014;3:1–7.

70. American Geriatrics Society 2012 Beers Criteria Update Expert Panel. American Geriatrics Society updated Beers criteria for potentially inappropriate medication use in older adults. J Am Geriatr Soc 2012;60:616–31. http://dx.doi.org/10.1111/j.1532-5415.2012.03923.x.

71. Forman DE, Rich MW, Alexander KP, et al. Cardiac care for older adults: time for a new paradigm. J Am Coll Cardiol 2011;57:1801–10.

72. Beckett NS, Peters R, Fletcher AE, et al, HYVET Study Group. Treatment of hypertension in patients 80 years of age or older. N Engl J Med 2008;358:1887–98. http://dx.doi.org/10.1056/NEJMoa0801369.

73. Sardar P, Chatterjee S, Chaudhari S, et al. New oral anticoagulants in elderly adults: evidence from a meta-analysis of randomized trials. J Am Geriatr Soc 2014;62(5):857–64. http://dx.doi.org/10.1111/jgs.12799.

74. Mohanty BD, Looser PM, Gokanapudy LR, et al. Controversies regarding the new oral anticoagulants for stroke prevention in patients with atrial fibrillation. Vasc Med 2014;19(3):190–204.

75. Reuben DB. Medical care for the final years of life: "when you're 83, it's not going to be 20 years". JAMA 2009;302:2686–94.

76. American Geriatric Society Expert Panel on the Care of Older Adults with Multimorbidity. Patient-centered care for older adults with multiple chronic conditions: a stepwise approach from the American Geriatrics Society: American Geriatrics Society Expert Panel on the Care of Older Adults with Multimorbidity. J Am Geriatr Soc 2012;60(10):1957–68. http://dx.doi.org/10.1111/j.1532-5415.2012.04187.x.

77. Emanuel EJ, Emanuel LL. Four models of the physician-patient relationship. JAMA 1992;267(16):2221–6.

78. O'Malley AS, Carrier ER, Docteur E, et al. Policy options to encourage patient-physician shared decision making. National Institute for Healthcare Reform; 2011. Available at: https://www.ecri.org/Documents/2011_TA_Conf/Resources/Policy_Options_to_Encourage_Patient-Physician_Shared_Decision_Making(National_Institute_for_Health_Care_Reform).pdf.

79. O'Connor AM, Bennett CL, Stacey D. Decision aids for people facing health treatment or screening decisions. Cochrane Database Syst Rev 2011;(10):CD001431. http://dx.doi.org/10.1002/14651858.CD001431.pub2.

80. American Geriatrics Society Expert Panel on the Care of Older Adults with Multimorbidity. Guiding principles for the care of older adults with multimorbidity: an approach for clinicians. J Am Geriatr Soc 2012;60(10):E1–25. http://dx.doi.org/10.1111/j.1532-5415.2012.04188.x.

81. Smith AK, Williams BA, Lo B. Discussing overall prognosis with the very elderly. N Engl J Med 2011;365:23.

82. Lim E. Patients' perspective in the surgical decision-making process. Thorac Surg Clin 2012;22:539–43.

83. Yourman LC, Lee SJ, Schonberg MA, et al. Prognostic indices for older adults: a systematic review. JAMA 2012;307(2):182–92.

84. Lee S, Smith AK, Widera E, et al. Eprognosis: estimating prognosis of elders. Available at: http://eprognosis.ucsf.edu. Accessed June 12, 2014.

85. Social security administration actuarial life table. Available at: http://www.ssa.gov/OACT/STATS/table4c6.html. Accessed June 12, 2014.

86. American College of Surgeons National Surgical Quality Improvement Program. Surgical risk calculator. Available at: http://riskcalculator.facs.org/. Accessed June 12, 2014.

Rehabilitation of the Geriatric Surgical Patient

Predicting Needs and Optimizing Outcomes

Walter L. Biffl, MD[a,b,*], Susan E. Biffl, MD[c,d]

KEYWORDS

- Geriatric • Rehabilitation • Surgery • Geriatric rehabilitation • Functional outcome
- Functional assessment • Frailty

KEY POINTS

- Geriatric surgical and trauma patients have a high likelihood of requiring institutionalization after discharge from acute care hospitalization, and this can be predicted by frailty.
- Standard assessment tools for functional status are important for communication and documentation of outcomes.
- The rehabilitation team has many members and offers many services with an overarching goal of optimizing functional status.
- Rehabilitation can be offered in multiple venues and the rehabilitation team is expert at identifying the most appropriate venue for each patient.
- More studies are needed to determine the optimal therapeutic interventions to improve functional outcomes in geriatric surgical patients.

INTRODUCTION: SCOPE OF THE PROBLEM

Geriatric patients, defined as those age 65 years or older, comprise approximately 13% of the population of the United States, but account for one-third of inpatient and outpatient surgical procedures.[1] Elderly patients undergoing major surgery or sustaining trauma often cannot be discharged home from the hospital. In a prospective study of 223 geriatric patients undergoing major surgery requiring postoperative intensive care unit (ICU) care, 30% required institutional care, such as nursing home

[a] Department of Surgery, Denver Health Medical Center, 777 Bannock Street, MC 0206, Denver, CO 80204, USA; [b] Department of Surgery, University of Colorado Denver School of Medicine, Denver, CO, USA; [c] Department of Orthopedic Surgery, Denver Health Medical Center, 777 Bannock Street, Denver, CO 80204, USA; [d] Department of Physical Medicine and Rehabilitation, University of Colorado Denver School of Medicine, Denver, 13001 E 17th Pl, Aurora, CO 80045, USA
* Corresponding author. Department of Surgery, 777 Bannock Street, MC 0206, Denver, CO 80204.
E-mail address: walter.biffl@dhha.org

(NH), skilled nursing facility (SNF), or rehabilitation unit (RU).[2] Joseph and colleagues[3] found that of 200 consecutive geriatric trauma patients, just 92 (46%) were discharged home; 5 (3%) died, 49 (25%) were transferred to a RU, and 54 (27%) to a SNF. Thus, rehabilitation is a major issue facing geriatric surgical patients. This article explores issues surrounding rehabilitation of the geriatric surgical patient.

PREDICTING THE NEED FOR REHABILITATION

Many large database studies have concluded that advanced age independently predicts adverse surgical outcomes in procedures ranging from major gastrointestinal resections to thyroid surgery.[4,5] However, that numerous centers report excellent outcomes for surgery in even the very elderly (eg, pancreatic resection in octogenarians[6]) suggests it is not simply age that affects outcomes.

A growing body of literature has addressed the issue of physiologic, rather than chronologic, age as a predictor of outcomes. Several clinical assessment tools have been used to assess physiologic status. In recent years a large body of surgical literature has focused on quantifying the degree of physiologic impairment, summarized as a frailty index (FI).

Frailty

Frailty has in the past been considered synonymous with disability (often a result of frailty), comorbidity (often a cause of frailty), or advanced old age (often a coincidence with frailty). Fried and colleagues[7,8] promulgated a standardized definition for frailty in 2001 (**Table 1**). Conceptually, the definition is based on five characteristics: (1) shrinking (unintentional weight loss), (2) weakness, (3) poor endurance/exhaustion, (4) slowness, and (5) low activity level. FIs have been developed to quantify frailty. The FI is calculated by counting an individual's deficits in health (eg, symptoms, signs, disabilities, comorbidities, laboratory data, electrocardiographic abnormalities) and dividing by the total number of deficits assessed.[9] Several FIs have been published, and some

Table 1 Characteristics of frailty and their definitions, based on data collected in the Cardiovascular Health Study	
Characteristic	**Definition**
Shrinking	Unintentional weight loss $\geq$10 lb or $\geq$5% body weight in prior year
Weakness	Grip strength (kg) in lowest quintile of Cardiovascular Health Study data[a]
Poor endurance	"Exhaustion" (self-reported)[b]
Slowness	15 ft walking time in lowest quintile[c]
Low activity	Kcal expended/week (self-reported)[d]

Frailty is defined as the presence of three or more criteria; "prefrailty" is defined by the presence of one or two criteria.
  [a] Stratified by gender and BMI. Men: BMI $\leq$24, grip strength $\leq$29 kg; BMI 24.1–28, grip strength $\leq$30 kg; BMI >28, grip strength $\leq$32. Women: BMI $\leq$23, grip strength $\leq$17 kg; BMI 23.1–26, grip strength $\leq$17.3 kg; BMI 26.1–29, grip strength $\leq$18 kg; BMI >29, grip strength $\leq$21.
  [b] Asked "How often in the last week did you feel either: (a) I felt that everything I did was an effort; or (b) I could not get going?" Subjects answering "a moderate amount of the time (3–4 days)" or "most of the time" categorized as frail.
  [c] Stratified by gender and height. Men: $\leq$173 cm, $\geq$7 seconds; >173 cm, $\leq$6 seconds. Women: $\leq$159 cm, $\geq$7 seconds; >159 cm, $\leq$6 seconds.
  [d] Stratified by gender, based on short version of Minnesota Leisure Time Activity Questionnaire activity scale: men, <383 kcal/wk; women, <270 kcal/wk.

interesting facts emerge. First, elderly individuals accumulate health deficits at a consistent rate of about 0.03 per year.[10] Second, there seems to be a consistent submaximal limit on the accumulation (ie, an individual can only possess about two-thirds of the health deficits assessed).[10] Most importantly, from study to study, although various FIs contain different types and different numbers of deficits, the higher the FI, the more vulnerable the individual is to adverse outcomes (ie, the FI is strongly associated with morbidity, institutionalization, and mortality).[9] Searle and colleagues[9] offered a list of 40 deficits (**Table 2**) and presented a standard procedure for creating an FI, suggesting that an FI can be created for use with any dataset.

Frailty and outcomes

Frailty has been found to be superior to age alone in predicting outcomes following trauma. In a prospective cohort study of 250 geriatric trauma patients, Joseph and colleagues[11] found that patients with frailty were more likely to suffer in-hospital complications (odds ratio, 2.5) and adverse discharge disposition, defined as death

Table 2
List of 40 variables included in the Frailty Index

Variable	Cut-Point (Point Value)
Need help with...bathing, dressing, getting in/out of chair, walking around house, eating, grooming, toileting, up/down stairs, lifting 10 lbs, shopping, housework, meal preparation, medication, finances; lost >10 lbs past year; stayed in bed >half a day due to health in past month; cut down on usual activity in past month	Yes (1)/no (0)
High blood pressure, heart attack, congestive heart failure, stroke, cancer, diabetes, arthritis, chronic lung disease	Yes (1)/suspect (0.5)/no (0)
Feel...everything is an effort, depressed, not happy, lonely, trouble getting going	Most of time (1)/some time (0.5)/rarely (0)
Self-rating of health	Poor (1)/fair (0.75)/good (0.5)/very good (0.25)/excellent (0)
How health has changed last year	Worse (1)/better or same (0)
Walk outside	<3 d (1)/$\geq$3 d (0)
Mini Mental State Exam	<10 (1)/11–17 (0.75)/18–20 (0.5)/20–24 (0.25)/>24 (0)
Peak flow (L/min)	[a]M $\leq$340; F $\leq$310
Shoulder strength (kg)	[a]M $\leq$12; F $\leq$9
BMI	<18.5 or $\geq$30 (1)/25–<30 (0.5)
Grip strength (kg)	[a]M $\leq$29 if BMI $\leq$24, $\leq$30 if BMI 24.1–28, $\leq$32 if BMI >28 F $\leq$17 if BMI $\leq$23, $\leq$17.3 if BMI 23.1–26, $\leq$18 if BMI 26.1–29, $\leq$21 if BMI >29
Usual pace walk 20 ft (s)	[a]>16
Rapid pace walk 20 ft (s)	[a]>10

Abbreviations: BMI, body mass index; F, female; M, male.
[a] Defines deficit.
From Searle SD, Mitnitski A, Gahbauer EA, et al. A standard procedure for creating a frailty index. BMC Geriatr 2008;8:24.

or discharge to SNF (odds ratio, 1.6). The investigators defined frailty as an FI greater than 0.25 using the FI assessment tool of Searle and colleagues.[9] All five patients who died in the study had frailty. Age was not independently associated with any of the primary outcome measures. In a subsequent study, the same investigative group[3] performed an analysis of all the variables in the FI of Searle and colleagues[9] and selected the 15 with the strongest association with an unfavorable discharge; they called these items the Trauma-Specific Frailty Index (**Table 3**). The Trauma-Specific Frailty Index was validated in a prospective study of 200 geriatric patients.[3] In all age groups, Trauma-Specific Frailty Index greater than 0.27 predicted unfavorable discharge; no other factor was significantly associated with unfavorable discharge.

Other Assessment Tools

Although geriatric patients can safely undergo major surgery, it is helpful and the responsibility of clinicians to counsel patients and their families on the expected course and outcomes of various alternatives. The ability to be discharged home after surgery is an important outcome to patients, and patients want to know the likelihood of that outcome. To that end, Hyder and colleagues[12] have derived and validated a tool to predict returning home after surgery (**Fig. 1**). The calculator is simple, based on only five questions, and was validated across multiple cohorts of surgical patients. As an example, an 80-year-old patient with insulin-dependent diabetes who is undergoing urgent or emergent surgery has a score of 37 and thus a 60% to 70% chance of requiring skilled services before returning home, even if previously living independently at home.

An even simpler assessment was proposed by Jones and colleagues.[13] Patients undergoing elective cardiac or colorectal surgery were asked if they had suffered a fall in the previous 6 months. One-third of the cohort of 235 patients had fallen, and falls were significantly associated with complications, readmissions, and institutionalization. This held true for colorectal and cardiac surgical patients (**Table 4**). Overall, if a patient had fallen three or more times in the previous 6 months, the risk of complications was 100%. This seems to be a simple means of assessing risk.

ASSESSING OUTCOMES

The goal of rehabilitation is to optimize a patient's functional status from a physical, cognitive, and psychological standpoint. In discussing rehabilitation, it is important to use standardized outcome assessments. There are several such tools available. Ardolino and colleagues[14] divided outcome measures following trauma into four subgroups: (1) functional, reflecting basic functioning and activities of daily living (ADL); (2) quality of life (QOL), including general health and satisfaction; (3) return to work, maintenance of education, and social dependency; and (4) patient experience. Although most would agree that the patient experience is an important metric, there is little to no standardization of patient experience assessment or benchmarks for rehabilitation of the geriatric surgical patient. Return to work and maintenance of education are not optimal metrics in geriatric rehabilitation because there can be many reasons why an individual does not return to his or her previous job or schooling, and geriatric patients are by definition beyond conventional retirement age. The Adult Social Care Outcomes Toolkit includes measures of social interaction; however, this is not widely used or reported. Moreover, such measures are generally included in other assessments. Consequently, the most widely used and reported outcome measures are functional measures and QOL assessments.

Table 3
The 15-item Trauma-Specific Frailty Index

Comorbidities	
Cancer history	
Yes	1
No	0
Coronary heart disease	
Myocardial infarction	1
Coronary artery bypass grafting	0.75
Percutaneous coronary intervention	0.5
Medication	0.25
No medication	0
Dementia	
Severe	1
Moderate	0.5
Mild	0.25
None	0
Daily activities	
Help with grooming	
Yes	1
No	0
Help managing money	
Yes	1
No	0
Help doing household work	
Yes	1
No	0
Help toileting	
Yes	1
No	0
Help walking	
Wheelchair	1
Walker	0.75
Cane	0.25
None	0
Health attitude	
Feel less useful	
Most time	1
Sometimes	0.5
Never	0
Feel sad	
Most time	1
Sometimes	0.5
Never	0
Feel effort to do everything	

(continued on next page)

Table 3 (continued)	
Most time	1
Sometimes	0.5
Never	0
Falls	
Most time	1
Sometimes	0.5
Never	0
Feel lonely	
Most time	1
Sometimes	0.5
Never	0
Function, sexually active	
Yes	1
No	0
Nutrition, albumin	
<3	1
>3	0

From Joseph B, Pandit V, Zangbar B, et al. Validating Trauma-Specific Frailty Index for geriatric trauma patients: a prospective analysis. J Am Coll Surg 2014;219:10–8; with permission.

Functional Outcome Assessment

Most of the literature on functional independence measures in geriatric surgery patients is based on either trauma or hip fracture surgery. Measuring functional outcomes is critical to quality improvement, and there are several ways that functional outcomes can be assessed. Three common assessments of overall function are the Barthel Index, the Functional Capacity Index (FCI), and the Functional Independence Measure (FIM).

Barthel Index

The Barthel Index, introduced in 1965, assesses independence in physical ADLs across 10 items, primarily related to self-care and mobility.[15] It was the major functional outcome assessment tool used in the United States until it was improved and ultimately supplanted by the FIM. It has been used most extensively to monitor functional changes in stroke patients receiving inpatient rehabilitation, and is still in use in some countries in a modified version.[16]

Functional Capacity Index

The FCI was designed to measure the reduced capacity to perform tasks considered important for everyday living.[17] It involves assessment of 10 different dimensions reflecting structurally independent aspects of function, with between three and seven levels of function identified for each dimension. It was targeted for use in trauma outcomes research and validated in 1240 blunt trauma patients. The FCI compared favorably with the Sickness Impact Profile and the 36-Item Short Form Health Survey (SF-36), discriminating better among patients according to the presence and severity of traumatic brain injury.[17] The FCI addresses physical and cognitive function only; it does not assess psychosocial well-being.

Scoring Your Discharge Destination						Your Score
How old are you?	20-39	40-49	50-59	60-69	70-79	80 or older
(POINTS)	0	4	8	12	16	20
Is your surgery elective surgery or not?	Elective		Not elective			
(POINTS)	0		8			
How independent are you for daily activities?	Independent		Partially dependent		Totally dependent	
(POINTS)	0		11		15	
Where were you living or being treated before surgery?	Home		Acute care facility		Nursing home	
(POINTS)	0		7		27	
What is your ASA Performance Status?	I or II		III	IV	V	
(POINTS)	0		9	17	30	

Circle the points that apply to you. Add them up to determine your score. Find your score on the figure.

Elective surgery means you came into the hospital for surgery on the same day and were not admitted beforehand to get "tuned up."
Independent means you require no assistance for bathing, feeding, toileting, dressing or transfer. Totally depdendent means that you require assistance with each of these tasks. Partially depdendent patients are neither totally independent nor totally dependent.
An acute care facility includes another hospital or emergency department or similar place where sick patients are diagnosed and treated.
Your ASA Performance Status would correspond to the following examples. If you have questions, ask your surgeon or anesthesiologist.

I or II Patients with no or only mild systemic disease. The majority of patients fall into this category.
    -You have hypertension, which is well controlled
    -You have diabetes which is controlled with oral medications only
III Patients with severe systemic disease. Some patients will be included in this category.
    -You have asthma that requires daily medications including occasional symptomatic treatments
    -You have diabetes which is poorly controlled or requires insulin therapy
IV Patients with severe systemic disease that is a constant threat to life. Few patients fall into this category.
    -You have asthma requiring daily medications including frequent symptomatic treatments or a recent hospitalization
    -You have diabetes which is poorly controlled, requires insulin therapy or for which you have had a complication such as vision loss or amputation
    -You have had heart disease that severely limits your ability to perform regular activities
V Patients who are moribund, or near death, for whom death is almost certain without surgery. Very few patients fit this category.

A

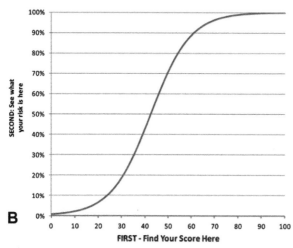

Fig. 1. Home discharge prediction calculator. (*A*) Example of the home calculator to predict home discharge. (*B*) Risk of not going straight home: comparing risk score and risk of not being discharged. (*From* Hyder JA, Wakeam E, Habermann EB, et al. Derivation and validation of a simple calculator to predict home discharge after surgery. J Am Coll Surg 2014;218(2):232; with permission.)

Table 4
Postoperative adverse outcomes related to having fallen in the previous 6 months

	Colorectal		Cardiac	
	Fallers	Nonfallers	Fallers	Nonfallers
Patients, N	29	52	49	105
Complications (%)	17 (59%)	13 (25%)	19 (39%)	16 (15%)
30-day readmission (%)	5 (19%)	2 (4%)	11 (23%)	8 (8%)
Institutionalization (%)	14 (52%)	3 (6%)	29 (62%)	33 (32%)

Data from Jones TS, Dunn CL, Wu DS, et al. Relationship between asking an older adult about falls and surgical outcomes. JAMA Surg 2013;148:1132–8.

Functional Independence Measure

The FIM is the most widely accepted functional assessment measure in use in the rehabilitation community.[18] The FIM is comprised of 18 items, grouped into two sub-scales (**Table 5**). The items are scored from 1 to 7; thus, the total score may range from 18 to 126. The FIM has consistently demonstrated good interrater reliability and valid-ity, and is an excellent tool for detecting changes during rehabilitation; however, there is a ceiling effect that limits its utility for long-term follow-up.[19] Another issue is that it does not address participation or activity elements (eg, return to work, relationships, social interactions) considered critical to outcomes and a measure of the burden of the disability.[18] The Functional Assessment Measure was developed as an adjuvant to the FIM. It was designed for brain-injured patients to address areas not covered by the FIM, such as behavioral, communication, and community functioning measures.[18] Although the Functional Assessment Measure may be more sensitive in identifying changes during rehabilitation, it is not used widely in reports of long-term outcomes.

Quality of Life Assessment

The patient's self-assessment of general health and satisfaction is a powerful outcome measure, and is the standard means of measuring health-related QOL. However, geri-atric patients may not provide accurate self-assessments. Magaziner and col-leagues[20] indicate that 40% of hospitalized geriatric patients are unable to provide accurate information. Even when able to address questions of functional status, geri-atric patients may underreport disability because of cognitive impairment, lack of self-awareness, or simply minimizing their functional limitations. Proxy reports can provide invaluable information, but should be compared with patient self-reports. Magaziner and colleagues[20] found that proxies tended to report more disability than the subjects

Table 5 Functional Independence Measure	
Motor Subscale	**Cognition Subscale**
Eating	Comprehension
Grooming	Expression
Bathing	Social interaction
Dressing upper body	Problem solving
Dressing lower body	Memory
Toileting	
Bladder management	
Bowel management	
Transfers: bed/chair/wheelchair	
Transfers: toilet	
Transfers: bathtub/shower	
Locomotion: walking/wheelchair	
Locomotion: stairs	

Each item is scored on a scale from 1 to 7: 7 = complete independence; 6 = modified indepen-dence, requires use of a device but no physical assistance; 5 = supervision, requires standby assistance, verbal prompting, or help with setup; 4 = minimal assistance, performs greater than 75% of task but requires hands-on assistance; 3 = moderate assistance, performs 50%–75% of task; 2 = maximal assistance, performs 25%–49% of task; 1 = total assistance.

Data from Nichol AD, Higgins AM, Gabbe BJ, et al. Measuring functional and quality of life out-comes following major head injury: common scales and checklists. Injury 2011;42:281–87.

themselves, and that discordance varied by specific function (eg, incontinence was reported more frequently by proxies than by patients). Weinberger and colleagues[21] compared self-reports with proxy reports and found that concordance was good in rating IADLs, as long as their Folstein mental state score was greater than or equal to 24 out of 30 (ie, not cognitively impaired).

36-Item Short Form Health Survey
The most commonly used measure of QOL is the SF-36. This survey originated from the Rand Corporation's health insurance experiment questionnaire, which contained 108 items.[22] Although the original instrument was sensitive and valid, its length made it impractical for general use. The SF-36 contains 36 items representing eight dimensions of health: (1) physical functioning (10 questions), (2) social functioning (two questions), (3) physical role limitations (four questions), (4) emotional role limitations (three questions), (5) mental health (five questions), (6) vitality (four questions), (7) pain (two questions), and (8) general health (five questions). One question addresses health changes or transition, and does not fit in any domain.[23] A shorter version, the SF-12, is less burdensome. It has been validated in trauma patients, but is not widely used at this time.[24]

Activities of daily living
As individuals age, their functional status inevitably declines. The Katz Index of Independence in Activities of Daily Living,[25] commonly referred to as the Katz ADL, is an excellent instrument to assess functional status in terms of the patient's ability to perform self-care tasks independently. The Katz ADL Index assesses independence in the six functions of bathing, dressing, toileting, transferring, continence, and feeding. Scoring 1 for a "Yes" and 0 for a "No," a score of 6 indicates full function, 4 indicates moderate impairment, and 2 or less indicates severe functional impairment. The ADL instrument is most meaningful when baseline measurements from the premorbid state are compared with subsequent measures. Although the Katz ADL Index is sensitive to changes in declining health status, it is limited in its ability to measure small increments of change seen in the rehabilitation of older adults.

Instrumental activities of daily living
In contrast to ADLs, instrumental ADLS (IADLs) are not necessary for fundamental functioning, but are necessary to live independently in a community. They include telephoning, shopping, food preparation, housekeeping, laundry, taking transportation, taking medications, and handling finances. The list of ADLs and IADLs is contained in **Table 6**. Buurman and colleagues,[26] in a literature review, found a great deal of variability in measuring ADLs and IADLs in elderly patients, and in the definitions of functional decline. This is problematic in interpreting literature comparatively.

Table 6 Activities of daily living and instrumental activities of daily living	
Activities of Daily Living	**Instrumental Activities of Daily Living**
Bathing	Using the telephone
Dressing	Shopping
Toileting	Food preparation
Transferring	Housekeeping
Continence	Laundry
Eating	Mode of transportation
	Responsibility for own medications
	Ability to handle finances

THE REHABILITATION PROCESS

The proliferation of geriatric RUs in the United States was catalyzed by the trial of Rubenstein and colleagues,[27] in which frail elderly inpatients assigned to a geriatric RU enjoyed a shorter hospital length of stay (LOS); were less likely to be discharged to an NH and had shorter NH LOS; and had better functional status and morale, fewer hospital readmissions, and lower mortality compared with standard care. As the population ages, more and more geriatric patients are candidates for rehabilitation. It is important to understand the process, including the timing, participants, techniques, goals, and expectations. Making good use of rehabilitation resources is facilitated by an appreciation for how disability occurs and the mechanisms by which rehabilitation is effective. This knowledge leads to understanding which specific rehabilitation services might best be provided, where to provide them, and by whom.

The Rehabilitation Team

Multidisciplinary care is the cornerstone of rehabilitation, because there are a myriad of health-related and contextual factors in a complex interaction that must be addressed in a coordinated fashion. The rehabilitation team in a RU is usually led by a physical medicine and rehabilitation specialist (physiatrist), but in some units the primary medical provider may be a neurologist, orthopedic surgeon, geriatrician, physician assistant, or nurse practitioner. The physiatrist has expertise in the entire rehabilitation process. He or she provides medical care, particularly emphasizing promotion of function, avoidance of polypharmacy, and optimization of nutrition. The physiatrist also has expertise in managing pain and spasticity, and prescribing appropriate prosthetics and orthotics. Other team members include nurses, therapists (physical, occupational, speech/language, hand, and recreation), dieticians, orthotists, prosthetists, psychologist/psychiatrists, and social workers.

Rehabilitation Interventions

Geriatric surgical patients may be disabled by acute and/or chronic health issues, and personal and environmental factors. Surgical and medical interventions target the health issues, whereas rehabilitation interventions are designed to address all of the covariates that impact the patient's well-being.

The rehabilitation process begins with an extensive assessment of the patient. The Comprehensive Geriatric Assessment (CGA) is a multidisciplinary assessment of medical, functional, and psychosocial issues including functional capacity (ADLs, IADLs), fall risk, cognition, mood, polypharmacy, social support, financial concerns, and goals of care. Additional components include nutritional status, continence, vision, hearing, dentition, sexual function, living situation, and spirituality. The depth of the assessment depends on the availability and expertise of team members. Ideally, geriatric surgical or trauma patients are cared for in an environment that provides appropriate resources. The CGA is performed by a physician (physiatrist or geriatrician), nurse practitioner, or physician assistant, along with a nurse and social worker; other team members include physical and occupational therapists, nutritionists, pharmacists, psychiatrists, psychologists, dentists, audiologists, podiatrists, and opticians as needed. Questionnaires for the patient or surrogates are helpful; however, the clinician must be cognizant of the potential inaccuracies reflected in patient and surrogate questionnaires. Geriatric patients may underreport disability because of cognitive impairment, lack of self-awareness, or simply minimizing their functional limitations.[20,21]

Once the assessment is completed, it is important to educate patients and families regarding options for rehabilitation and to set expectations. The patients and their families will have their own expectations, and these should be reconciled with the rehabilitation team's assessment of current status and what the rehabilitation team can reasonably expect to achieve. In general, rehabilitation interventions include the components discussed next.[28]

Physical therapy
The physical therapist assesses strength, range of motion, gait, and mobility; and designs and oversees an exercise program to improve or maintain fitness and maximize mobility, within medical limitations. The program may be designed to improve parameters, such as muscle strength, endurance, flexibility, and motor control. They have a role in recommending assistive devices and environmental modification (see later). The physical therapist also may provide treatments for pain.

Occupational therapy
The occupational therapist evaluates ADLs particularly related to self-care skills, and creates interventions to improve these skills. The therapist also performs home safety evaluations and designs a plan for environmental modification; he or she may fabricate splints and treat upper extremity deficits, including recommendations for assistive technology.

Speech and language therapy
A speech and language pathologist (speech therapist) can use clinical observation, radiographic, and/or endoscopic studies to clarify the nature of dysphagia and fine-tune recommendations. Treatment of dysphagia may be directed by the speech and language pathologist individually or in collaboration with a nutritionist and/or occupational therapist. Speech therapists also provide interventions for cognitive disabilities, often in concert with occupational therapy and neuropsychology.

Assistive devices
In the United States as of 1997, 14% of people older than the age of 65 used mobility devices: 3% required a wheelchair or scooter, 5% a walker, and 10% used a cane.[29] Patients recovering from major surgery or trauma are even more likely to require use of some form of mobility assistance. The rehabilitation team assesses the need for and prescribes assistive devices. Medicare pays for such "durable medical equipment" but there are guidelines that must be followed, including justification by a physician, nurse practitioner, or physician assistant. The rehabilitation team also assesses the need for and prescribes bathroom assistive devices (eg, toilet, bathtub, or shower modifications). Prosthetics (artificial devices that replace a body part) and orthotics (external devices applied to a body segment to support or improve its function) are also the purview of the rehabilitation team. The rehabilitation team assesses the patient's overall function to provide the optimal intervention to support a patient. For example, a severely debilitated geriatric amputee may do better with a wheelchair than with a prosthesis. A physiatrist, physical therapist, and prosthetist are typically be involved in that decision. Orthoses may be prefabricated, or they may be custom-fitted by an orthotist or an occupational therapist.

Environmental modification
An important intervention of the rehabilitation team is to modify the patient's environment to minimize impairment and enhance "accessibility." Occupational therapists have particular expertise in barriers to self-care and challenging cognitive

situations. Physical therapists are particularly helpful with mobility impairments and equipment.

Pain management
The rehabilitation team invariably deals with pain, particularly in geriatric surgical and trauma patients. Primary modalities include analgesic medications, heat and cold application, and transcutaneous electrical nerve stimulation.

Social work
Social workers can help patients cope with a disability, assist with accessing resources, and address challenging family dynamics. They play a major role in navigating the transition from acute care to postdischarge rehabilitation.

Psychology
Rehabilitation psychologists assess and address emotional and behavioral concerns to support patients and families; they can also assist with cognitive deficits.

Rehabilitation nursing
The role of the rehabilitation nurse cannot be minimized. The nurse must provide medical care and monitoring for deterioration, and at the same time provide encouragement and support for the process and maintain the schedule of therapies.

REHABILITATION SETTINGS

Rehabilitation therapy can be delivered in a wide variety of settings across the continuum of care, from the ICU to RU and even the patient's home. The nature of the services differs based on the environment and the patient's medical condition, but the focus on the goal of maximizing function is consistent. To optimize outcomes, the rehabilitation process should ideally begin in the preoperative phase. The American College of Surgeons and American Geriatric Society promulgated recommendations for preoperative assessment of geriatric surgical patients, which encompass a wide breadth of health issues (**Box 1**).[1] Essentially the American College of Surgeons and American Geriatric Society recommends an assessment akin to the CGA, with interventions designed to improve the patient's health status before undergoing surgery.

Rehabilitation Therapy During Acute Hospitalization

Whereas Rubenstein and colleagues[27] showed the benefits of geriatric RUs, rehabilitation therapies have been provided during acute medical care. In a prospective randomized trial, Landefeld and colleagues[30] assigned general medical patients to a unit designed to help older patients achieve or maintain self-care independence. Key elements of the unit included environmental enhancements (uncluttered hallways, handrails, large clocks), patient-centered and customized care emphasizing independence, discharge planning with the goal of return to home, and intensive review of medical care to avoid errors. Compared with those receiving routine care, patients assigned to the special unit had greater improvement in their ability to perform ADLs at the time of discharge, and were less likely to be transferred to a long-term care facility. Much of the literature on early mobilization and other interventions comes from populations of medical patients, but surgical patients also may benefit. In a recent study, a program of intensive physiotherapy was designed for trauma patients hospitalized at a level I trauma center.[31] The two additional 30-minute physiotherapy sessions per day resulted in improved mobility and patient satisfaction compared with their standard regimen of a single session per day. However, the investigators found

---

Box 1
Preoperative assessment of the geriatric surgical patient

In addition to conducting a complete history and physical examination of the patient, the following assessments are strongly recommended:

- Assess the patient's **cognitive ability** and **capacity** to understand the anticipated surgery.
- Screen the patient for **depression**.
- Identify the patient's risk factors for developing postoperative **delirium**.
- Screen for **alcohol** and other **substance abuse/dependence**.
- Perform a preoperative **cardiac** evaluation according to the American College of Cardiology/American Heart Association algorithm for patients undergoing noncardiac surgery.
- Identify the patient's risk factors for postoperative **pulmonary** complications and implement appropriate strategies for prevention.
- Document **functional status** and history of **falls**.
- Determine baseline **frailty** score.
- Assess patient's **nutritional status** and consider preoperative interventions if the patient is at severe nutritional risk.
- Take an accurate and detailed **medication history** and consider appropriate perioperative adjustments. Monitor for **polypharmacy**.
- Determine the patient's **treatment goals** and **expectations** in the context of the possible treatment outcomes.
- Determine patient's **family** and **social support system**.
- Order appropriate preoperative **diagnostic tests** focused on elderly patients.

From Chow WB, Rosenthal RA, Merkow RP, et al. Optimal preoperative assessment of the geriatric surgical patient: a best practices guideline from the American College of Surgeons National Surgical Quality Improvement Program and the American Geriatrics Society. J Am Coll Surg 2012;215:453–66; with permission.

---

no difference in destination once therapeutic goals had been achieved, LOS, or QOL measures.

Advances in critical care management, and surgical care in general, have resulted in more survivors of critical illness. Unfortunately, many of them suffer prolonged disability. To counter overall disability, and weakness in particular, early physical and occupational therapy with mobilization in the ICU has been promoted. Noting that in the 1960s and 1970s, mechanically ventilated patients were routinely mobilized, investigators have bemoaned the current ICU with heavily sedated, bedridden patients.[32] Several studies have demonstrated safety with early mobilization of critically ill patients. One prospective randomized clinical trial found that patients having early physical and occupational therapy enjoyed better functional outcomes when discharged, shorter duration of delirium, and more ventilator-free days.[33]

Clearly, the hospitalized patient's ability to participate in physical or occupational therapy are predicated on the patient's cognitive, hemodynamic, musculoskeletal, and pain status. Although the optimal combination of interventions may not have been identified, it seems that some therapy is better than none in the acute care setting. Furthermore, even if patients cannot participate in therapy, involvement of rehabilitation team members is vital for discharge planning in any patient for whom there is concern about the ability to return home.

Rehabilitation After Acute Hospitalization

A common concern of surgeons and their patients is determining the most appropriate level of care after the patient has recovered from the surgical procedure. Fewer than half of severely injured patients are discharged home,[3] and one-third of elective surgical patients requiring admission to the ICU then require some form of institutional care.[2] There are a variety of venues to consider, which vary in the types and intensity of therapies available, the medical and nursing support, and reimbursement. The options for venues include inpatient RUs, long-term acute care hospitals, SNFs, home health, and outpatient therapies. The options and considerations are summarized in **Table 7**. Factors involved in the decision-making are numerous and discussed next.

Medical diagnoses

Under Centers for Medicare and Medicaid Services guidelines, eligibility for admission to an RU may be contingent on diagnoses. Specifically, 60% of patients admitted to a facility for rehabilitation must have 1 of 13 diagnoses. Multiple trauma diagnoses are

Table 7
Options for post–acute care rehabilitation

Site	Physician Coverage	Nursing Coverage	Therapy Services	Medicare Coverage
Inpatient rehabilitation unit	Physician evaluation at least 5 d/wk; physician available 24 h/d, 7 d/wk	24-h care	Physical, occupational, speech therapy available; patient must need at least two therapy services and must receive therapy at least 3 h/d, 5 d/wk	Days 1–20: 100% Days 21–100: 80% plus copayment Days >100: 0%
Skilled nursing facility	Physician evaluation within 2 wk of admission, plus every 30 d; physician available in emergencies	24-h care	Physical and occupational therapy available; at least one session per day	Same as rehabilitation unit
Long-term acute care facility	Physician evaluation as needed for medical conditions; physician available 24 h/d	24-h care	Physical and occupational therapy available	Same as rehabilitation unit
Home therapy	Physician referral; physician recertification every 60 d	Home health nurse	Physical, occupational, and speech therapy available	1–3 visits per week for 1–3 wk; 1 visit per week with registered nurse, daily home health aid
Outpatient therapy	Physician referral; physician recertification every 30 d	None	Physical, occupational, and speech therapy available	May be limitations in number of visits per year

on the list, including spinal cord injury, brain injury, major multiple trauma, amputation, femur and fracture, and burn injury. However, the average general surgical patient does not have one of those or the remaining diagnoses (stroke, congenital deformity, neurologic disorders, arthritides, vasculitides, osteoarthritis, or hip or knee replacement). If an RU already has too many patients without proper diagnoses, it limits access to more patients without those diagnoses. Early involvement of the rehabilitation team is important to establish options and align everybody's expectations: patient, family, surgeon, and rehabilitation team.

Medical stability
Even if a patient has an appropriate diagnosis, their medical stability may dictate eligibility for a specific level of care. Patients with active significant medical problems are more appropriate for an RU or long-term acute care facility where staff physicians are available, rather than a skilled nursing care or home care where physician presence is not as consistent.

Functional status
Current and premorbid functional status also impact the decision on placement, because RUs require 3 hours of active participation in therapy each day. Patients with appropriate diagnoses may simply not be able to participate.

Cognition
Candidates for RUs must have the cognitive capacity to follow simple commands, and sufficient recall to enable learning.

Tolerance and motivation for therapy
A patient who refuses therapy during acute care hospitalization is unlikely to be accepted for rehabilitation services, because participation is mandatory. However, this factor can potentially change rapidly as the patient recuperates, pain subsides, nutrition improves, and medications are adjusted.

Types of services needed
To be accepted into an RU, a patient must have needs for at least two types of services (eg, physical and occupational therapy).

Psychosocial factors
These include patient and family preference and geographic location, but also the patient's ability to stay safe, and for the caregivers to be safe, in treating the patient.

Third-party reimbursement
This is a major consideration for many patients. Medicare has a "prospective payment" system, whereby a predetermined amount of coverage is provided for various diagnoses. For example, payment for rehabilitation services after a stroke is 12 to 14 days; alternatively, the same patient would be eligible for 20 days at 100% coverage, and 80 more days at 80% coverage, in a SNF. The patient's medical condition, service needs, and other factors impact the decision. Social workers generally work with patients and families on these decisions. Home health care has several restrictions, including the requirement that a patient actually needs "skilled" services, and not just a home health aid. Medicaid also covers rehabilitation services but the coverage varies from state to state. Outpatient rehabilitation services are covered by Medicare as "fee-for-service," but the total number of visits for all conditions is limited. In 2012, the limits were $1870 per year for physical therapy plus speech therapy, and an additional $1870 per year for occupational therapy.

OUTCOMES FOLLOWING REHABILITATION

There is a paucity of literature on rehabilitation of the geriatric surgical patient. Rubenstein and colleagues[27] reported dramatic benefits associated with rehabilitation services in 1984. Subsequent studies have included meta-analyses with the finding that inpatient multidisciplinary rehabilitation programs were associated with improvement in all outcomes at discharge, including better functional status, decreased NH admission, and reduced mortality.[34] Recently, Joseph and colleagues[35] reported that FIM scores increased by an average of 29 points from the time of admission to the rehabilitation facility and discharge. Unfortunately, geriatric rehabilitation services are not prevalent outside of the Veterans Affairs system.

REALITIES OF REHABILITATION

There are several issues that complicate the concept of providing rehabilitation services to all geriatric surgical patients, and expecting improved outcomes.

Financing

Most rehabilitation facilities require payment for services. The rules regarding reimbursement are outlined previously. Many surgical patients do not have 1 of the 13 diagnoses that Centers for Medicare and Medicaid Services requires for admission; many more patients do not have the required finances to pay for the services. Thus, many patients are not eligible for admission. It is important to consult the rehabilitation team early, because an appropriate setting should be identified and to allow enough time for prior authorization of payment by insurers.

Home Support

The ability of a geriatric patient to function independently at home often requires support from other family and friends in the home. This is a barrier for many patients.

Functional Status

Patients who have severely compromised functional status from injuries may never return to functional independence in their previous living situation, regardless of rehabilitation interventions.

GAPS IN KNOWLEDGE

There is a paucity of literature pertaining to rehabilitation of geriatric surgical and trauma patients; moreover, there are few high-quality, prospective randomized clinical trials of like individuals that provide evidence for management strategies. Indeed, a Cochrane Collaboration review of literature on rehabilitation of elderly patients in long-term care concluded that rehabilitation efforts may be beneficial, reducing disability with few adverse events. However, effects are quite small and may not be broadly applicable. Furthermore, there is insufficient evidence to make conclusions regarding the most appropriate and beneficial interventions, improvement sustainability, or cost-effectiveness.[36]

Specific interventions have simply not been studied to a degree necessary to recommend "best practices." The Geriatric Trauma Committee of the American Association for the Surgery of Trauma was created in 2012 and as of August 2014 is preparing a White Paper addressing gaps in knowledge in managing geriatric trauma patients, and recommending a research agenda.

REFERENCES

1. Chow WB, Rosenthal RA, Merkow RP, et al. Optimal preoperative assessment of the geriatric surgical patient: a best practices guideline from the American College of Surgeons National Surgical Quality Improvement Program and the American Geriatrics Society. J Am Coll Surg 2012;215:453–66.
2. Robinson TN, Wallace JI, Wu DS, et al. Accumulated frailty characteristics predict postoperative discharge institutionalization in the geriatric patient. J Am Coll Surg 2011;213:37–44.
3. Joseph B, Pandit V, Zangbar B, et al. Validating trauma-specific frailty index for geriatric trauma patients: a prospective analysis. J Am Coll Surg 2014;219:10–8.
4. Kurian AA, Wang L, Grunkemeier G, et al. Defining "the elderly" undergoing major gastrointestinal resections: receiver operating characteristic analysis of a large ACS-NSQIP cohort. Ann Surg 2013;258:483–9.
5. Abraham CR, Ata A, Carsello CB, et al. A NSQIP risk assessment for thyroid surgery based on comorbidities. J Am Coll Surg 2014;218:1231–7.
6. Hatzaras I, Schmidt C, Klemanski D, et al. Pancreatic resection in the octogenarian: a safe option for pancreatic malignancy. J Am Coll Surg 2011;212:373–7.
7. Fried LP, Tangen CM, Walston J, et al. Frailty in older adults: evidence for a phenotype. J Gerontol A Biol Sci Med Sci 2001;56:M146–56.
8. Fried LP, Borhani NO, Enright P, et al. The cardiovascular health study: design and rationale. Ann Epidemiol 1991;1:263–76.
9. Searle SD, Mitnitski A, Gahbauer EA, et al. A standard procedure for creating a frailty index. BMC Geriatr 2008;8:24. http://dx.doi.org/10.1186/1471-2318-8-24.
10. Rockwood K, Mitnitski A. Frailty in relation to the accumulation of deficits. J Gerontol A Biol Sci Med Sci 2007;7:722–7.
11. Joseph B, Pandit V, Zangbar B, et al. Superiority of frailty over age in predicting outcomes among geriatric trauma patients. JAMA Surg 2014;149(8):766–72. http://dx.doi.org/10.1001/jamasurg.2014.296.
12. Hyder JA, Wakeam E, Habermann EB, et al. Derivation and validation of a simple calculator to predict home discharge after surgery. J Am Coll Surg 2014;218:226–36.
13. Jones TS, Dunn CL, Wu DS, et al. Relationship between asking an older adult about falls and surgical outcomes. JAMA Surg 2013;148:1132–8.
14. Ardolino A, Sleat G, Willett K. Outcome measurements in major trauma: results of a consensus meeting. Injury 2012;43:1662–6.
15. Mahoney FI, Barthel DW. Functional evaluation: the Barthel Index. Md State Med J 1965;14:61–5.
16. Shukla D, Devi BI, Agrawal A. Outcome measures for traumatic brain injury. Clin Neurol Neurosurg 2011;113:435–41.
17. MacKenzie EJ, Sacco WJ, Luchter S, et al. Validating the functional capacity index as a measure of outcome following blunt multiple trauma. Qual Life Res 2002;11:797–808.
18. Nichol AD, Higgins AM, Gabbe BJ, et al. Measuring functional and quality of life outcomes following major head injury: common scales and checklists. Injury 2011;42:281–7.
19. Hall K, Bushnik T, Lakisic-Kazazic B, et al. Assessing traumatic brain injury outcome measures for long-term follow-up of community-based individuals. Arch Phys Med Rehabil 2001;82:367–74.
20. Magaziner J, Zimmerman SI, Gruber-Baldini AL, et al. Proxy reporting in five areas of functional status: comparison with self-reports and observations of performance. Am J Epidemiol 1997;146:418–28.

21. Weinberger M, Samsa GP, Schmader K, et al. Comparing proxy and patients' perceptions of patients' functional status: results from an outpatient geriatric clinic. J Am Geriatr Soc 1992;40:585–8.
22. Ware JE, Brook RH, Williams KN, et al. Conceptualization and measurement of health for adults in the health insurance study. Model of health and methodology, vol. 1. Santa Monica (CA): Rand Corporation; 1980 (Publication No R-1987/1-HEW).
23. Kopjar B. The SF-36 health survey: a valid measure of changes in health status after injury. Inj Prev 1996;2:135–9.
24. Kiely JM, Brasel KJ, Guse CE, et al. Correlation of SF-12 and SF-36 in a trauma population. J Surg Res 2006;132:214–8.
25. Katz S, Ford AB, Moskowitz RW, et al. Studies of illness in the aged: the index of ADL: a standardized measure of biological and psychosocial function. JAMA 1963;185:914–9.
26. Buurman BM, van Munster BC, Korevaar JC, et al. Variability in measuring (instrumental) activities of daily living functioning and functional decline in hospitalized older medical patients: a systematic review. J Clin Epidemiol 2011;64:619–27.
27. Rubenstein LZ, Josephson KR, Wieland GD, et al. Effectiveness of a geriatric evaluation unit: a randomized clinical trial. N Engl J Med 1984;311:1664–70.
28. Hoenig H, Kortebein PM. Overview of geriatric rehabilitation: program components and settings for rehabilitation. Available at: www.UptoDate.com. Accessed July 25, 2014.
29. Kaye HS, Kang T, LaPlante MP. Mobility device use in the United States. Disability statistics report no. 14. Washington, DC: National Institute on Disability and Rehabilitation Research, U.S. Department of Education; 2000.
30. Landefeld CS, Palmer RM, Kresevic DM, et al. A randomized trial of care in a hospital medical unit especially designed to improve the functional outcomes of acutely ill older patients. N Engl J Med 1995;332:1338–44.
31. Calthorpe S, Barber EA, Holland AE, et al. An intensive physiotherapy program improves mobility for trauma patients. J Trauma Acute Care Surg 2014;76:101–6.
32. Needham D. Mobilizing patients in the intensive care unit: improving neuromuscular weakness and physical function. JAMA 2008;300:1685–90.
33. Schweickert WD, Pohlman MC, Pohlman AS, et al. Early physical and occupational therapy in mechanically ventilated, critically ill patients: a randomized controlled trial. Lancet 2009;373:1874–82.
34. Bachmann S, Finger C, Huss A, et al. Inpatient rehabilitation specifically designed for geriatric patients: systematic review and meta-analysis of randomized controlled trials. BMJ 2010;340:c1718. http://dx.doi.org/10.1136/bmj.c1718.
35. Joseph B, Pandit V, Aziz H, et al. Rehabilitation after trauma; does age matter? J Surg Res 2013;184:541–5.
36. Crocker T, Forster A, Young J, et al. Physical rehabilitation for older people in long-term care (review). Cochrane Database Syst Rev 2013;(2):CD004294. http://dx.doi.org/10.1002/14651858.CD004294.pub3.

End-of-Life Care of the Geriatric Surgical Patient

Jacob Peschman, MD[a], Karen J. Brasel, MD, MPH[b],*

KEYWORDS

- Do not resuscitate • Palliative care • Hospice • Care conferences • Goals of care
- End-of-life • Surgical ethics • Palliative surgery

KEY POINTS

- End-of-life care is a broad topic that can only be done successfully with defined goals of care, familiarity with symptom management, and comfort in addressing personal and professional ethics.
- Terminal illnesses include a broad range of diseases and lengths of survival, providing unique challenges to the managing surgeon.
- Basic understanding of the differences between health care power of attorneys, advanced directives, and do not resuscitate, as well as the roles of palliative care and hospice care are key to engaging in discussions with patients and families.
- Management includes controlling pain, dyspnea, nausea and vomiting, and understanding the role and difficulties of discussing palliative surgery with patients and their families.

INTRODUCTION

"Cure sometimes, treat often, comfort always"

—Hippocrates

Nature of the Problem

Everyone dies; there is really nothing more certain in life. Despite this, a patient's preparation for the care that he or she desires at the end of life and open discussion with his or her physician remain suboptimal. In 1991, the Patient Self Determination Act was passed, which required health care institutions to inform and document patients of their rights in regards to medical decision making, including refusal of life-sustaining therapies or cardiopulmonary resuscitation. Yet, in the mid 2000s, reported rates of pre-established do not resuscitate (DNR) orders were as low as 15% in patients undergoing surgery.[1] Although surgeons are often involved in the

[a] Department of Surgery, Medical College of Wisconsin, 9200 W. Wisconsin Avenue, Suite 3510, Milwaukee, WI 53226, USA; [b] Department of Surgery, Oregon Health and Science University, Mailcode L223, Portland, OR 97239, USA
* Corresponding author.
E-mail address: brasel@ohsu.edu

Surg Clin N Am 95 (2015) 191–202
http://dx.doi.org/10.1016/j.suc.2014.09.006
0039-6109/15/$ – see front matter © 2015 Elsevier Inc. All rights reserved.

surgical.theclinics.com

care of patients with life-threatening illnesses, additional single-institution reviews found surgical services lagging behind medical services in establishing DNR documentation for patients at the time of their death, with approximately 60% with established DNR orders in the records and 75% with physician-documented discussions about DNR status.[2] Surgical services also took nearly twice as long (9.8 vs 5.1 days) to establish DNR status after admission than their medical colleagues.

Comfort in discussing end-of-life care and decision making affects nearly every surgeon. The breadth of diseases managed in surgical specialties encompasses everything from cancer to dementia and trauma. This highlights not only why it is important for surgeons to be comfortable with end-of-life discussions but also why the discussions can be so difficult. Not all deaths occur the same way, especially in geriatric patients. Although patients with malignancies may suffer a slow decline, trauma patients may have been highly functional prior to their terminal traumatic event. **Fig. 1** represents the varying trajectories of functional decline geriatric patients experience.[3–5] Therefore, discussion as early as possible with patients and their families about end-of-life wishes when the patient is most functional is the ideal time to establish goals of care no matter what the disease process.

GOALS OF CARE

"It is much more important to know what sort of a patient has a disease than what sort of a disease a patient has"

—*William Osler*

How to Discuss Goals of Care

The most important aspect of providing good end-of-life care to geriatric patients is having a discussion about the goals of care. Ideally, this conversation should include patients when they are at their normal functional status, as this allows them to express their desires as well as establish which family members they wish to be involved in the dialogue. Several recommendations may facilitate goals of care discussions:

- Preface goals of care and DNR discussions with statements that these talks occur with all patients. This can help to diffuse patient perception that the physician believes their condition may be imminently life threatening.
- When possible, discussion points should be readdressed over multiple visits in the office or hospital to address any questions the patients may develop between encounters or changes in their wishes.

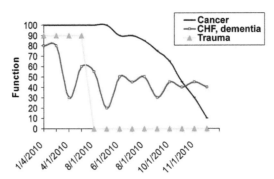

Fig. 1. The trajectory of functional decline in geriatric patients. CHF, congestive heart failure. (*Data from* Refs.[3–5])

- Allow adequate time for the discussion.
- Although one does not need a definitive answer regarding DNR status at the first meeting, one should be formally established and documented as early as possible.
- Provide expectations with evidence as to the likelihood of a patient having a meaningful outcome after cardiopulmonary resuscitation. This will differ based on comorbidities and primary disease process.
- It is acceptable to give a recommendation after listening to a patient's goals.
- The physician should provide patients and family with the institution's advance directive forms and adequate instructions for having them become part of their medical record.

Family Care Conferences

Involvement of a patient's family and friends in end-of-life discussions is critical. At the very end of life, patients will often be unable to express their own wishes, and family members will be their surrogates, making decisions on their behalf. Family care conferences can allow teams of physicians and associated health care providers to speak in an open group forum, limiting miscommunication or perceptions of mixed messages from different providers. These can occur in the outpatient, inpatient, or intensive care unit (ICU) settings, and can be used as either updates on overall care plans such as in treatment sequencing in cancer care, or to address specific decision points such as withdrawal of life-sustaining therapies. Similar principles apply to any setting.[6]

- One physician or specialty team should be established as the facilitator prior to the meeting. This person or team should be involved in deciding which consulting services, nurses, therapists, social workers, and other team members should. should attend.
- Health care providers should review the patient's record immediately prior to the meeting to ensure they are up to date on current conditions and plans. If there are multiple providers attending a meeting, these providers should communicate with each other prior to the meeting to prevent any disagreements in care plans from arising during the meeting.
- A location should be chosen that is of adequate size, limits noise or extraneous distractions, and has access to needed accessories (ie, a white board for drawing pictures, computer monitors to view imaging studies). It may be helpful to have tissue boxes or additional smaller rooms available nearby for family members who can become emotionally overwhelmed by the content of the discussion.
- The meeting facilitator should start with prompting introductions of all persons present in the room including their role in the patient's care or relationship to the patient.
- A family spokesman should be established if at all possible. This person should be the legal decision maker as established by local laws and regulations or the patient's documented health care power of attorney (HCPOA). In the absence of a HCPOA, this may be a source of disagreement in families. Using the family meeting to help establish which person will be the HCPOA is helpful.
- Establish goals for the conference (eg, information sharing and DNR determination).
- Have family members explain their understanding of the patient's condition and course. Allow them the time to complete their thoughts without interrupting or injecting additional details or corrections.

- Relay any additional information the family about which the family was unaware of or unclear. Use repetition and allow questions to be asked. Answer the questions as specifically as possible. Acknowledge uncertainty when it exists.
- Avoid the temptation to give too many specific medical details.
- Review prognosis, the expected course, and next steps as clearly as possible.
- Acknowledge emotions and allow for periods of silence.
- Ask open-ended questions when exploring fears and concerns. Make sure to phrase questions in terms of what the patient would want or what the patient would want the family to do.
- Make it clear that care is never withdrawn even when life-sustaining therapies may be discontinued. The family should know that their doctors and nurses are still treating the patient even if the focus of the treatment has changed.
- Make recommendations when appropriate.
- Recap discussions at the end and make sure all of the initial goals were accomplished. This is a good time to summarize and clarify any specific decisions that were made.
- Remember, not all members of the family may agree on treatment plans, so not all decisions may be made at this time. It will be up to the discretion of the facilitating physician to decide if any critical urgent decisions need to be made prior to ending the meeting or if there is time for the family to discuss things further.
- Establish follow-up planning for the meetings. For short-term follow up in ICU settings for example, a specific time can be set, often in the next 48 to 72 hours. In the outpatient setting time, frames will be longer. Telephone contact or specific interactions with the HCPOA may be necessary based on work or other conflicts.
- Provide a means for the family to contact providers with follow-up questions. This may also be a good time to select a family spokesperson to prevent multiple different family members from expecting specific one-on-one conversations with the care team, especially in the setting of family discord or disagreement.

Defining Advanced Directive, Health Care Power of Attorney and Do Not Resuscitate

There is some confusion concerning the differences between living wills, advance directives, HCPOAs and DNRs. Some of the confusion stems from the terms being used interchangeably in situations; some from the fact that different states will have different specific details surrounding each as they are applicable within that state. The best reference for a surgeon will be his or her specific institution's and state's policies although each will be briefly described here.[7]

Advanced directives, advanced health care directives, medical directives, or living wills

These are defined as: "written expression of how you want to be treated in certain medical circumstances." They can address any number of scenarios in specific or general terms. Examples include use of feeding tubes, mechanical ventilation, discharge to nursing facilities, and desire for cardiopulmonary resuscitation or intubation.

Health care power of attorney, power of attorney for health care, health care proxy, durable medical power of attorney, health care surrogate

These are defined as "durable power of attorney specifically designed to cover medical treatment." These designate a person who will make decisions on the patient's behalf, although they do not specify what decisions should be made. If these have not been specifically designated by the patient with written documentation, and the patient is deemed not decisional or not capable of making his or her decisions, state laws will dictate the hierarchy by which this person is appointed. Certain states have no hierarchy and instead defer to the morally relevant agent. If no person exists, can be contacted, or it is felt by the health care team that there is conflicting interest in the legal designee, a court-appointed designee may be necessary. Involvement of an institution's ethics board may be helpful in this situation.

Do not resuscitate
A DNR is a physician order regarding the implementation of therapy if the patient were to suffer from cardiopulmonary arrest.

The details of a DNR order are institution dependent and may specifically differentiate between aspects of cardiopulmonary resuscitation (chest compressions vs chemical code) and intubation. Each physician should refer to his or her own institutions policies for specifics.

Community DNR orders are available in most states and can provide the patient with some form of identifying documentation, such as a wristband, that identifies his or her DNR status should they suffer an out-of-hospital/health care facility arrest. Discussion of DNR status should be documented in the patient's medical record at the time of discussion, whether he or she chooses to be DNR or not.

The American College of Surgeons do not resuscitate policy
There remains some confusion and disagreement in the medical community as to DNR status in patients undergoing surgery. The American College of Surgeons (ACS)[8] and American Society of Anesthesiologists (ASA)[9] have both published position statements in regards to the continuation of a DNR order in the perioperative period. Highlights include

- Institutional policies that automatically enforce or cancel pre-existing DNR orders do not sufficiently support a patient's right to self-determination
- Physicians should discuss and document DNR status with the patient or surrogate decision maker prior to proceeding with a planned operation
- Options include suspending the DNR for a defined time frame in the perioperative period, continuing the DNR in the perioperative period, and limiting specific interventions (such as chest compressions but not intubation) in the perioperative period
- If a health care provider has an ethical or professional conflict with the patient's advance directive, an alternative provider should be recruited

Futility policies
There will be times when despite open conversations with patients and their family members, there will be disagreement with their physicians over the use of certain life-sustaining therapies. Medical futility refers to the concept of appropriateness of medical treatment.[10]

Quantitative utility defines a situation in which the expected intervention has a small (typically <1%) chance of success. Qualitative utility defines a situation in which the quality of the benefit will be exceedingly poor.

Texas and California at present have state-wide futility policies, while the majority of the country relies on individual institutional policies. Physicians are not legally, ethically, or professionally required to provide any medically futile therapy as defined by the standards of the medical community. Some institutional policies will also allow physicians to enact DNR orders even if the family of the patient is in disagreement, although utilizing good communication and intuitional ethics consultation, usually involving a nonbiased third party to facilitate discussion should be employed first.

Defining Palliative Care and Hospice

Although many palliative care specialists are involved in facilitating hospice care, the two are distinct from one another despite the terms commonly being used interchangeably. Palliative care is "an approach which improves the quality of life of patients and their families facing life-threatening illness, through the prevention, assessment and treatment of pain and other physical, psychosocial, and spiritual problems." It provides a framework for managing whole patients with debilitating problems, even when death may not be imminent, to include chronic incurable illnesses and those that threaten life.

Hospice is a focus on care rather than cure for patients with chronic and terminal illnesses. Although the philosophy is similar to palliative care, dedicated hospice services are defined by Medicare. This is to dictate reimbursement for services that include coverage of medications, physicians, nursing care, and providing a nursing facility or home environment for a patient who has been deemed by the treating physician as having a life expectancy of 6 months or less due to their medical condition(s).

SYMPTOM MANAGEMENT

> "The quality of life is more important than life itself"
> –Alexis Carrel

Even when death is inevitable, there is still much to be done in the care of patients. Managing pain, nausea, dyspnea, and other symptoms at the end of life can provide a quality of life and dignity to dying patients that may mean more to them and their families than invasive and difficult treatments with little chance of cure. Familiarity with basic principles of symptom management can greatly improve the care provided at the end of life.

Pain

Pain is the subjective unpleasant sensory and emotional experience that occurs as a result of actual or potential damage to a patient's tissue.[11,12] It may be difficult to manage because of the complex interplay of many factors. Involvement of multimodal therapies and palliative care physicians experienced in managing these symptoms can be extremely helpful. Basic concepts for the inpatient or outpatient settings are highlighted:

- Due to the subjective nature of pain, standardized pain scales can be helpful in managing pain. Establishing goal treatment levels allows the patient and surgeon to work toward acceptable control in situations in which complete resolution of pain is not possible.
- Many patients may not be able to verbalize their pain experience. Carefully observe for symptoms including grimacing, asking for nonspecific help, guarding, rocking, fidgeting, changes in behavior such as aggression, withdrawal, or food refusal, crying, and increased or decreased sleep.
- Opioids remain a mainstay of pain management.
  - Dose escalation is appropriate to control pain. Consider percentage of baseline use dose increases ranging from increases of 25% to 50% for moderate pain to 100% to 200% for palliative pain management at the end of life.
  - Tolerance refers to the need for dose escalation. Dependence refers to development of symptoms of withdrawal. True dependence is rare when opioids are used in end-of-life care, and therefore fear of developing dependence should not prevent appropriate dose escalation when needed.

- ○ The use of long-acting and short-acting opioids may be useful. For patients unable to take oral medications, evaluate for alternate administration methods including intranasal and transdermal administration.
- ○ Opioid patient-controlled analgesia (PCA) devices allow a patient to administer physician-dictated dose of medications. Many times providing this control to the patient provides additional psychological benefits. Also, in the palliative care setting, family members can be allowed to administer doses in patients who are no longer able to do so themselves, providing them similar benefits in countering feelings of helplessness.
- Utilizing nonopioid pain medications as part of multimodal therapy gives physicians additional options.
  - ○ Consider scheduling nonsteroidal anti-inflammatory medications and acetaminophen.
  - ○ Antidepressants such as selective serotonin reuptake inhibitors (SSRIs) can be a useful adjunct if initiated early in the treatment course, as they can take several weeks to have an effect.
  - ○ Treatment of neuropathic pain with gabapentin or pregabalin can be done in conjunction with use of opioids and can be especially helpful in patients with nerve involvement of tumors or fractures.
- Anxiety can compound pain in many patients. Benzodiazepines can provide analgesic benefits.
- Regional therapies such as nerve blocks or ablations may be helpful in some malignancies. Utilizing multispecialty pain services can often identify patients who may benefit.
- Treatment strategies should focus on the patient experience. Frequently reassessing adequacy of pain control and adjusting in a timely manner are mandatory.
- Route of medication administration is important. Re-establishment of intravenous access is painful, and intramuscular administration is also painful. Oral administration may not be possible. Sublingual and subcutaneous administration of morphine is equally effective as more commonly used routes and is much easier on the patient.
- Discussion with family members and caregivers about their impressions of adequacy of pain control can also be helpful in adjusting therapy.

Dyspnea

Dyspnea can be particularly distressing to patients and family members of those suffering from multiple disease processes including fluid overload due to heart or renal failure, pneumonia, advanced pulmonary disease, or those with rib fractures. It is a common complaint in end of life care and should be addressed in a similar goal-directed manner as pain control.[13,14]

Minimizing fluid intake, including the use of scopolamine patches to dry up secretions, is an important primary treatment.

Opioids are the most commonly employed treatment used in management of dyspnea; they have the double effect of depressing respiratory effort. Benzodiazepines and SSRIs can relieve some of the distress associated with feelings of dyspnea.

Oxygen administration has long been used in the management of dyspnea, although Cochrane reviews have not definitively demonstrated benefit. The use of continuous positive airway pressure (CPAP) and bi-level positive airway pressure ventilation can be considered in patients with significant dyspnea and respiratory muscle weakness, although they provide only temporary support and often are more uncomfortable for the patient to wear than the benefit derived.

As with pain management, frequent reassessment to provide adequate therapy adjustments should be central in patient management strategies.

Terminal Weaning

Many patients may be on a ventilator at the end of their life. Advanced directives and HCPOA decisions to respect the wishes of the patients may ultimately lead to the withdrawal of mechanical ventilation. If terminal weaning is desired, there are strategies that can ease the process and reduce any discomfort experienced by the patient. Consideration should also be given to minimizing family discomfort, as watching a loved one struggle to breathe is extremely disconcerting.

Efforts should be taken to minimize fluid intake, as described previously. Sedation should be used based on clinical indicators such as tachypnea and tachycardia. Opioids should be initiated prior to initiation of terminal weaning and escalated as needed to prevent dyspnea.

Terminal extubation involves removal of the endotracheal tube in a single step with premedication and rapid adjustments of opioids and sedatives as needed.

Terminal weaning involves step-wise and gradual reductions of oxygenation and ventilation. At each step the patient should be assessed for signs and symptoms of dyspnea with appropriate sedation and opioids provided. Weaning to a T-Tube or extubation can occur rapidly (<15 minutes) or gradually over hours with no evidence indicating a benefit.

Racemic epinephrine can be used for stridor following extubation. Monitor and ventilator alarms should be turned off during the process to avoid unnecessary distress to family members and staff members who are present.

Reported length of survival varies based on the underlying disease and degree of ventilator dependence, with times ranging from 2 minutes to several days and median times of several hours. Families should be counseled on this before the process is started to allow for appropriate emotional preparation.

Nausea and Vomiting

Nausea and vomiting are less common at the end of life in most disease processes than other symptoms previously discussed but can be very distressing to the patient. Treatment strategies should be based on specific reports of symptoms, making the effort to distinguish between dyspepsia, nausea, retching, vomiting, and regurgitating.[15]

It is important to exclude mechanical causes of nausea and vomiting, including bowel obstruction due to abdominal adhesions or advanced malignancy. In this case imaging with abdominal radiograph or computed tomography scans may be useful. If identified, risks and benefits of surgical and nonsurgical treatment should be discussed with the patient and family.

Dyspepsia can be the result of stress response, immobility, or pre-existing reflux disease. Management with proton pump inhibitors and H-2 blockers typically provides good success.

Regurgitation and emesis can be the result of gastric dysmotility or gastroparesis. This can be the result of other medications or because of malignancy. Promotility agents including metoclopramide, erythromycin, and antidopaminergic agents. Each has potential adverse effects and may require trial-and-error methods to determine which has the best affect for a specific patient.

Retching and nausea can be caused by dysfunction of the emetic pathway, a term used to refer to the central mechanisms of the perception of nausea. Treatments include medications previously listed, as well as benzodiazepines, steroids, and SSRIs.

Patients with malignant bowel obstructions may receive some benefit from octreotide to reduce gastrointestinal secretions from the intestines and pancreas contributing to discomfort.

Constipation can result from opioid use in many patients receiving end-of-life care and results in significant nausea and vomiting. Appropriate bowel regimens include stool softeners, bulking agents, and stimulants. Treatment should be guided to result in regular soft bowel movements to avoid discomfort. Suppositories can be considered if they are not too distressing to the patient.

Palliative Surgery

Surgeons may be asked to see patients with terminal illnesses to provide surgical therapies for palliation of different symptoms. In these patients, the previously discussed issues of perioperative DNR and adequate discussion of risks and benefits are crucial as operative complications may hasten the dying process.

When brought in for surgical consultation for palliative reasons, be sure to clarify the goals and expectations of the patient and family pertaining to the role of surgery. Unfortunately, many times the idea of surgery in advanced malignancies can confuse patients as being performed for possible cure. Adequate time for a thorough discussion is critical to avoid giving false hope.

Gastrostomy tubes are commonly suggested for geriatric patients. Clear indications for placement are necessary, which include both relief of obstruction and provision of nutrition. The benefit to patients with advanced dementia is questionable, and some studies indicate worse outcomes among patients.[16] If there is question as to appropriateness of placement or medical futility, ethics consultation should be obtained.

Surgical therapy for malignant bowel obstructions can be successful for some patients in relieving obstructive symptoms and re-establishing the ability to have oral intake but comes at the cost of significant mortality and prolonged hospitalizations.[17] Pleural catheters to drain malignant or persistent pleural effusions to relieve dyspnea can offer significant benefit to some patients.[13]

Utility of Electronic Medical Records and Order Sets

The transition of most health care institutions to the use of electronic medical records (EMRs) has multiple implications for end-of-life care. First, in theory, EMRs should increase the access to documented advanced directives and HCPOA documents to multiple providers in the system. Unfortunately, a recent review of advanced care EMR documentation in over 30,000 patients in California found that only 33% of patients with known advanced directives or HCPOAs had scanned copies of their documents accessible in the EMR.[18] Familiarity with an individual institution's documentation locations and processes for getting documents uploaded to the EMR is worth the effort. Having the discussion and documenting it are necessary, but having the legal documents available and uploaded as early as possible will allow all physicians and health care providers in a system to honor a patient's wishes.

An additional role of the EMR is developing order sets for use in palliative care and end-of-life situations. These can allow providers with less experience a quick, accessible, and standardized reference to help transitions the patient's treatment plan. Items can include placing appropriate consultations, common medications, and nursing orders to avoid overlooking key components that do not initially come to mind.

ETHICAL CONSIDERATIONS

"Ethics is nothing else than reverence for life"
                                                    —Albert Schweitzer

End-of-life care includes a host of ethical and moral issues beyond the scope of this article. However, 2 basic distinctions between commonly held misconceptions, of both patients and providers, are important. Understanding the difference between the concept of withdrawal and withholding and DNR and do not treat may not clarify any ethical or moral discrepancies, but should help patients develop a framework for them to develop their beliefs.

Withdrawal Versus Withholding

Withdrawal is defined as "the act of taking back or away something that has been granted or possessed."[19] Withholding is defined as "to hold back from action" or "to refrain from granting, giving, or allowing."[20]

The concept of taking something away is often more difficult to accept than never giving something in the first place. However, ethically and legally there is no difference when it comes to medical treatment. The goal of advanced directives and patient discussions with their HCPOA and physician is to prevent placing patients or HCPOAs in a situation where they are forced to make these decisions. However, especially in the ICU setting, where a significant proportion of people die every year, these decisions are common.

Early discussions with families and patients cannot be stressed enough, as specific interventions, especially intubation, hemodialysis, or the initiation of enteral or parenteral nutrition, become imminent. No escalation of therapy is a common philosophy that can be viewed by patients and some providers as a compromise. Therapies such as mechanical ventilation and nutrition are commonly continued while initiation of hemodialysis or vasopressors are more likely to be withheld.[21] Defining a specific end point or the length of time a specific therapy will be given at the beginning of treatment can help with treatment plans also.

Do Not Resuscitate Versus Do Not Treat

There is often a misconception that DNR signifies the end of medical treatment. This is untrue. As previously discussed, a DNR is simply a physician order that prevents the initiation of specific therapies in the event of cardiopulmonary arrest. As such, there are several facts about DNR that can be pointed out to patients and their families when having these discussions:

- A DNR order does not signify the end of treatment of any current medical condition.
- DNR is not reserved for the end-of-life. Many highly functional geriatric patients with reasonable life expectancies and varying medical conditions express their desire not to have heroic measures performed in the event of cardiopulmonary arrest.
- DNR does not exclude someone from treatment in the ICU, aggressive chemotherapy or surgical treatments, or even intubation for respiratory distress. However, the specifics of an institution's DNR policy should be part of the patient discussion, as the details of specific therapies (ie, chest compressions, vasopressors, or defibrillation) can be individually approved or declined at some institutions.

- A DNR order is not permanent. It can be discontinued or suspended at any time at the request of the patient or HCPOA. A change in DNR status should not be made without including discussion with the health care providers to explore the desires of these changes and clarify any questions.

SUMMARY

Patients and their families should never feel as if their doctors are giving up on them. Unfortunately, popular culture has associated terms like DNR with stopping treatment and palliative care with end-of-life care or hospice when there is nothing left to be done. Education, good communication, and compassionate care are a physician's only armaments against these misconceptions. Understanding end-of-life care terminology and goal-based treatment strategies for pain, dyspnea, and other unpleasant symptoms are needed for the physician to be able to take part in the care of patients and families in this important phase of their lives.

REFERENCES

1. Ewanchuk M, Brindley PG. Ethics review: perioperative do-not-resuscitate orders-doing 'nothing' when 'something' can be done. Crit Care 2006;10(4):219.
2. Morell E, et al. The do-not-resuscitate order: associations with advance directives, physician specialty and documentation of discussion 15 years after the Patient Self-Determination Act. J Med Ethics 2008;34(9):642–7.
3. Covinsky KE, et al. The last 2 years of life: functional trajectories of frail older people. J Am Geriatr Soc 2003;51(4):492–8.
4. Lynn J, Adamson DM. Living well at the end of life. Adapting health care to serious chronic illness in old age. Washington, DC: Rand Health; 2003.
5. Meier DE, Morrison RS. Autonomy reconsidered. N Engl J Med 2002;346(14): 1087–9.
6. Curtis JR, et al. The family conference as a focus to improve communication about end-of-life care in the intensive care unit: opportunities for improvement. Crit Care Med 2001;29(Suppl 2):N26–33.
7. Living wills, health care proxies, advance health care directives. 2014. Available at: http://www.americanbar.org/groups/real_property_trust_estate/resources/estate_planning/living_wills_health_care_proxies_advance_health_care_directives.html. Accessed July 6, 2014.
8. [ST-19] Statement on advance directives by patients: "do not resuscitate" in the Operating Room. 2013. Available at: http://www.facs.org/fellows_info/statements/st-19.html. Accessed June 28, 2014.
9. Ethical guidelines for the anesthesia care of patients with do-not-resuscitate orders or other directives that limit treatment. 2013. Available at: https://www.asahq.org/For-Members/Standards-Guidelines-and-Statements.aspx. Accessed June 28, 2014.
10. Cuezze JE, Sinclair CT. Medical futility. Fast facts and concepts. 2005; 136. Available at: http://www.eperc.mcw.edu/EPERC/FastFactsIndex/ff_136.htm. Accessed June 28, 2014.
11. Ruder S. 7 tools to assist hospice and home care clinicians in pain management at end of life. Home Healthc Nurse 2010;28(8):458–68.
12. Mularski R, et al. Pain management within the palliative and end-of-life care experience in the ICU. Chest 2009;135(5):1360–9.
13. Kamal A, et al. Dyspnea review for the palliative care professional: treatment goals and therapeutic options. J Palliat Med 2012;15(1):106–14.

14. Campbell M. How to withdraw mechanical ventilation: a systematic review of the literature. AACN Adv Crit Care 2007;18(4):397–403.
15. Glare P, et al. Treating nausea and vomiting in palliative care: a review. Clin Interv Aging 2011;6:243–59.
16. Candy B, et al. Enteral tube feeding in older people with advanced dementia: findings from a Cochrane systematic review. Int J Palliat Nurs 2009;15(8): 396–404.
17. Paul Olson T, et al. Palliative surgery for malignant bowel obstruction from carcinomatosis: a systematic review. JAMA Surg 2014;149(4):383–92.
18. Wilson C, et al. Multiple locations of advance care planning documentation in an electronic health record: are they easy to find? J Palliat Med 2013;16(9): 1089–94.
19. Definition of withdrawal. 2014. Available at: http://www.merriam-webster.com/dictionary/withdrawal. Accessed July 26, 2014.
20. Definition of withhold. 2014. Available at: http://www.merriam-webster.com/dictionary/withholding. Accessed July 26, 2014.
21. Morgan C, et al. Defining the practice of "no escalation of care" in the ICU. Crit Care Med 2014;42(2):357–61.

Index

Note: Page numbers of article titles are in **boldface** type.

Surg Clin N Am 95 (2015) 203–215
http://dx.doi.org/10.1016/S0039-6109(14)00193-5
0039-6109/15/$ – see front matter © 2015 Elsevier Inc. All rights reserved.

surgical.theclinics.com